The Well-Managed

Mental

Health

PRACTICE

The Well-Managed
Mental
Health
PRACTICE

*Your Guide to Building and Managing a
Successful Practice, Group, or Clinic*

DONALD E. WIGER

John Wiley & Sons, Inc.

Contents

Preface: The Business of Mental Health

This text is intended to serve several purposes, and is not simply a book on how to manage a mental health clinic. It goes to the next level by describing several problems one can encounter as a clinic director or manager either in private practice, as a clinic decision maker, or as someone aspiring to these positions. It also describes several of the nonclinical skills needed, both as a therapist and a clinic director or manager, to be successful in a private practice or clinic setting. It is written by a psychologist who has started successful practices and has worked in, managed, and owned both small and large mental health clinics.

Very little of the material taught in this text was learned in a book because most of the information hasn't been available in prior texts. Thus, there is no bibliography. Several fine texts are available describing how to start a mental health practice. This book includes the important aspects of starting a practice, but continues with instruction in management techniques, how to grow your business, and samples of clinic policies and procedures designed to conform to accreditation, third-party requirements, and sound business practices.

The bulk of the material in this text was learned from the school of hard knocks and through years of experience. Some of the lessons I have learned have been the result of very expensive setbacks, while others have been richly rewarding. Many of these difficult business or clinical judgments began with few or no guidelines or direction. The decisions I made turned out to be either gold mines or land mines.

When we think of gold mines we likely have visions of wealth, prosperity, success, good fortune, doing something correctly, or making the right decision. When someone says, "That decision was a gold mine," it was clearly a stellar decision. Gold mine decisions are usually difficult to make and may require the cost of extra effort and risk, but the end result can be a gold mine for the clinic and the career of the therapist. Results include such rewards as helping more clients, increased income, better service to clients, a successful audit, a low cost-benefits ratio, increased referrals, a positive reputation, feelings of fulfillment, a better working environment, increased income, decreased expenses, or a number of other positive indicators of success.

Land mines are quite the opposite. They may result in financial loss, harm to one's reputation, embarrassment, loss of clients, ethical complaints, loss of business, going out of business, or even leaving the field. They often represent what might seem right at the time or the quickest and easiest course of action. Or we may perform an action over a long period of time because we were misinformed or not educated in the topic. But in the end, these landmine decisions blow up in your face.

The reader will learn more than simply what is helpful or not helpful in clinical practice and management, but will also be given examples of several gold mine versus land mine decisions that could make or break one's practice, reputation, and sense of well-being. A primary goal of this text is to be a gold mine of information to its readers.

The text is organized in two units, Part A: Building a Practice, and Part B: Administrative and Documentation Procedures. Part A focuses on exploring the meaning of success as a therapist, in terms of customer service, increased business, positive employee relations, development of a professional reputation, priority setting, time management, and coping with stress. Part B deals with administrative and documentation issues that, if not learned, could lead to multifaceted problem areas clearly detrimental to the clinic and its leadership.

DEDICATION

This book is dedicated to Sirad Osman, the founder and director of New American Community Services in St. Paul, Minnesota. My experience with this organization has altered my ideas and feelings about the world. New American Community Services provides educational, medical, social, cultural, vocational, and psychological help to Somali and other West African refugees now living in Minnesota.

Every time I conduct an evaluation for one of their clients, my heart sinks as I am told of inhumane treatment, torture, a life of flight, loss of all possessions, and witnessing loved ones killed simply for being who they are. They moved to this country with a glimmer of hope that life would be different and they would be safe. However, many of the first-generation refugees simply do not, or cannot, get over the memories, scars, and sense of loss. New American Community Services is there to help.

American customs and religious practices are foreign to them—just about as unusual as their customs seem to us. Learning English is next to impossible when you live a life of fear, depression, and suffer from severe post-traumatic stress disorder. Some clients come into my office shaking, believing that I might be a government interrogator. It can be difficult to convince them otherwise. These evaluations have stretched my ability to empathize and demonstrate true compassion.

As a group they are a very kind and loving people, but many Americans look down on them because they receive public assistance and because they do not understand our language, our dominant religion, the concept of $1 + 1 = 2$, what a pair of pajamas is, or any of our customs or the way of life we take for granted.

Basic academic skills such as math, reading, and writing are not that important when there are no schools, there is no longer a place to call home, and you are fleeing for your life, often with no food. Let us welcome them, and others, who seek out our kindness for survival, safety, and a chance for their offspring to enjoy the same freedoms we take for granted. Many of the readers of this book are likely third- to fifth-generation Americans. Most of us are removed from the type of struggles that completely change one's life.

I admire their sense of community. These refugees typically

live in the same neighborhoods or in the same apartment complex as others from their culture. Many have no family here to help take care of them. They have no idea if their family survived. But their strong sense of community is like an informal social service agency. The stronger members shop, cook, clean house, and check on the weaker members. This sentiment is as strong as an American sense of family. We oftentimes say that blood is thicker than water. To these refugees, nothing is thicker than community.

http://www.newamericans.us

The Well-Managed

Mental
Health

PRACTICE

Part A

Building a Practice

Introduction

This introduction discusses therapists more than clinic management. Its purpose is to describe the type of therapist who does well in a management position. There are several skills and personality traits needed to effectively direct a mental health clinic. The basics are described in this chapter.

Graduate school for mental health professionals typically prepares students to diagnose and treat clients. Such skills are clearly necessary, but do not sufficiently prepare students for business success or management skills. This book teaches several skills that are not typically taught in graduate schools. Most of the lessons learned here are usually learned through trial and error. Hopefully the reader will be spared from some of the errors this author has made over the years.

There are myriad decisions a therapist must make when starting, maintaining, and managing a mental health clinic. Unless a therapist stays in contact with experienced colleagues for guidance and supervision, many of these executive decisions will be based on a hunch or intuition, rather than on training, supervision, and experience. These decisions (or even not being aware that decisions must be made) can easily lead to mismanagement or even going out of business. A clinic can quickly go from making a solid profit to being in the red due to a series of minor events. Being a good therapist clearly is not enough to stay in business, manage a clinic, or supervise others. This book discusses the skills necessary to not only stay in business or manage others, but also how to flourish in the field.

I have learned, over several years of hits and misses, a number of lessons regarding what works and what does not work when managing a mental health clinic, and the learning process continues. To complicate the matter, what worked one year may or may not work the next. We must be in touch with the pulse of this ever-changing field, but all too often become set in our way of doing things and do not see the world around us changing. The adage "If it works, don't change it," might make sense, but when the rules and procedures outside of your control change, you could be left behind or your practice become stagnant. A mark of a successful leader in the profession of mental health is the ability to be aware of and adapt to change. Although people may have difficulty dealing with change, it is inevitable. Not all change is good, but without change there can be no progress.

Often, what seems to be a good idea may not actually be at all helpful. There are many unwritten rules that are typically learned only by a series of positive and negative experiences. What feels or seems right isn't necessarily the best decision.

This text is not intended to focus solely on the mechanics of how to set up a private practice or manage a clinic. It goes beyond the "what to do" aspect to very specific "how to" and "how not to," behaviors. Many cautions will be given that were learned through very stressful and expensive experiences I have had directly or through supervising other professionals.

SUCCESS AS A THERAPIST

Mental health therapists enter the field for a variety of reasons, ranging from altruism to visions of wealth. The meaning of *success* as a mental health therapist has about as many connotations as the concept of happiness. Each of us has our own definition of success, so several possible aspects of success are discussed in this text. Therapists might view success in a number of ways, such as their commitment to helping clients, personal fulfillment, financial attainment, or a combination of factors. Our concept of success evolves throughout the years as we mature.

Some therapists fully devote their energy, time, and priorities to being a "helper." Those from an *others-orientation* show much genuine concern for their clients. Monetary gain means very little to them. Therapists who are extreme in this position typically work long hours and often see many clients free of charge or at a very low rate in order to meet the needs of others. When a client's bill is not paid, they are apt to let it go. However, they are likely to have problems meeting their own survival needs, and this may, eventually, cause them to become ineffective with clients.

A *self-oriented* therapist focuses on financial gain and self-interest. These persons enter the field for reasons such as feeling good about themselves when they help others, financial motivation, or any other reason that aids their own sense of gain. They typically make sound financial and business decisions and will likely be an asset in business matters. If monetary gain and self-aggrandizement are their first priority they will likely not be effective helpers.

Therapists functioning at either extreme, being selfless or selfish, are not likely to find success due to an excessive or insufficient sense of self. Both self-oriented and others-oriented therapists have specific skills that both help and hinder them from obtaining success in the field. There are also numerous additional skills that can increase any therapist's level of competence and success. These skills begin with procedures employed from the client's first phone call to the clinic. Success is clearly not one dimensional, and many different skills are needed to succeed no matter how it is defined.

Helping clients with their emotional needs, practicing in a professional manner, and making a good living creates a win-win situation for the therapist, the client, and the reputation of the profession. One can be caring, passionate, therapeutically effective, and make a very comfortable living in mental health. Therapists can learn to be well-rounded and avoid the extremes of being too self-oriented or too others-oriented.

This text does not intend to be a cookbook of instructions on how to be successful. Not only would this task be foolish, but it would also be impossible. However, this text can provide instruction in a number of areas where success is often measured or valued by mental health therapists. It is helpful for therapists in training or for therapists who want to develop or increase various clinic leadership skills.

WHAT DO SUCCESSFUL PEOPLE HAVE IN COMMON?

The word *success* is commonly defined in terms of achieving certain goals. However, each of us has different goals and views of what or who is successful. For example, one type of success as a therapist is attaining a desired level of achievement in the field. It is not uncommon to make statements such as, "She is (or is not) a very successful person." In mental health, whether success is achieved by helping others through life-changing therapy, being recognized in the field as an expert, being an excellent teacher, having a number of publications, being a good team player, having feelings of self-fulfillment, achieving financial goals, or any combination of these, it is highly valued.

We look up to people who we believe are successful. However, we might not respect those who openly boast of their own success. We tend to admire people who talk positively about other people's success but not their own. We doubt or distrust people claiming to be successful, but tend to believe those claims when others say they are successful. Success has a clear component of humility.

Vocational or career success is measured quite differently across the professions. In baseball, a player's number of home runs, hits, ability to catch, running speed, salary, and popularity are some of the components of success. An electrician's success might be measured by the number of jobs completed correctly, customer feedback, expertise, job stability, profit margins, or supervision abilities. A successful administrative assistant might be identified by business skills, efficiency, and social skills. Likewise, mental health therapists define a successful career by a different standard than other professions. Views of a successful therapist tend to focus on what they do, what they become, or some combination of these.

Globally, success may also be measured by such aspects as job or life satisfaction. However, this text focuses on specific components of a therapist's success, rather than on overall life satisfaction. Although the two might be related, it is possible to be professionally successful but lacking in life satisfaction.

LEARNING FROM PAST FAILURES

Success does not just happen. Most people experience a series of fortunate and unfortunate situations throughout their lives. The fortunate events may be positive experiences but have little to do with being successful. For example, a person winning the $100 million lottery is certainly fortunate, but is not necessarily successful. Success is multifaceted. It is not situational, nor is it achieved by attaining a single goal. It is the process of learning through one's victories and defeats.

Successful people might fail outwardly a number of times in their lives, but an inner drive to accomplish life goals drives them to continue reaching out. Few people would disagree that Abraham Lincoln was successful. However, he lost more elections than he won, he was not considered to be good looking, and he did not amass much wealth, but he goes down in history as one of America's greatest presidents. Successful people likely fail more than nonsuccessful people. But rather than repeating their failures or becoming defensive or defeatist, they learn from their mistakes. Making mistakes may get them down, but it does not keep them down; it motivates them to try something else and find what works. Failures in our lives lead to success if we treat them as learning tools, not endpoints. Do not be afraid to fail; it can lead to great success.

MOTIVATION AND DIRECTION

Motivation is a common denominator for successful people. People who are motivated are used to sometimes working long hours to finish a project, while others wouldn't think of paying a price that would interfere with their personal time. They do not procrastinate, but, rather, finish a project they are proud of in a timely manner.

They look at barriers as stepping stones, rather than as stumbling blocks. When they fail, they bounce back up with more determination, having benefited from learning what not to do the next time around.

Although motivation is necessary, it is not sufficient, in itself, for success. One must also have direction. Direction involves setting reasonable goals, having the means or ability to achieve them, sticking with them, and making alterations as needed. Simply being motivated, without direction, is a guaranteed road to failure or mediocrity. A highly motivated person who lacks direction is like having the world's faster racehorse, but letting it run around aimlessly in a field. Success finds motivated people who have proper direction.

BEING AN AVERAGE THERAPIST

It is remarkable how most people understand the word *average* as having negative connotations. There is nothing wrong or unusual about being an average therapist; however, few of us want to be considered as average. Notice the difference between the following two sentences: "Pat is an average therapist," and "The average therapist is both helpful to her clients and makes a comfortable living." Although each sentence contains the word *average,* the connotations differ. In the first sentence, Pat might not be flattered by being referred to as an average therapist. In the second sentence, the term *average* is fairly positive. Typically, a motivated person desires to be above average, not to be better than others, but rather to do well in the field. This book will be most helpful for those who desire or endeavor to become above average in a variety of areas pertaining to the business side of the mental health industry.

By definition, the word *average* denotes the level that describes most people in a given attribute. However, for some reason, being describes as average has negative connotations to many people. For example, consider a group of medical students in an Ivy League university. When they take a test, most of them will make an average score compared to the others in their class. Only a certain number will stand out in this highly intelligent group of people. Amongst themselves, most are "average," but before attending an Ivy League medical school, many of them may have been class valedictorians. The term *average* is a relative term compared to the reference group. An average therapist has much to be proud of. But, to be in management of other therapists, one must learn above average skills.

When referring to average therapists, the term is relative to other advanced degreed therapists. An average therapist will see about 20 to 25 clients per week, for about 6 to 10 sessions. A certain number of their clients will report that therapy was helpful, but certainly not all of them. An average therapist's income was about $60,000 to $80,000 annually in 2006. Overall, when considering a normal or bell-shaped curve, a certain amount of people will be very successful, some will be very unsuccessful, while most will experience normal careers as therapists. Although there is no need to rise beyond being average, there are those who choose to excel—but there is a price to pay.

DEFINING, MEASURING AND INCREASING ELEMENTS OF SUCCESS AS A THERAPIST

A normal curve of therapist attributes suggests that there are multiple behaviors by which a therapist's success may be measured. It is clearly possible to be successful in some areas, but not in others. For example, a therapist might have a very low income, but be very effective with clients, while the reverse may be true for another therapist. Which of the two is more successful? Of course, there is no clear answer. In a normal curve most people fall in the middle. Very few fall at the two extremes. This text teaches specific skills to increase one's ability to function at the upper end of the curve. Obviously, no therapist will want to excel in every area. For example, some people are more interested in having a higher income than others. Each individual views success through different lenses. This text attempts to teach the means to obtain success. Figure I.1 lists sev-

FIGURE I.I
Level of Attainment in Various Therapists' Attributes Possibly Suggesting "Success"

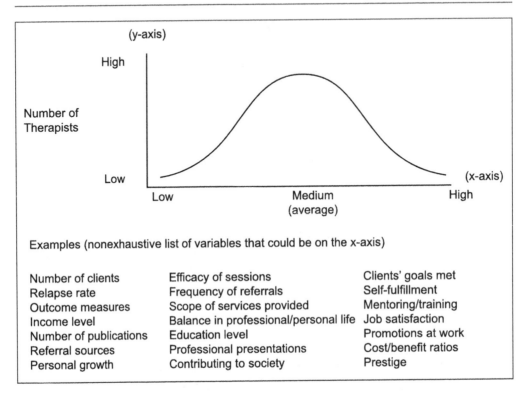

Examples (nonexhaustive list of variables that could be on the x-axis)

Number of clients	Efficacy of sessions	Clients' goals met
Relapse rate	Frequency of referrals	Self-fulfillment
Outcome measures	Scope of services provided	Mentoring/training
Income level	Balance in professional/personal life	Job satisfaction
Number of publications	Education level	Promotions at work
Referral sources	Professional presentations	Cost/benefit ratios
Personal growth	Contributing to society	Prestige

eral possible areas therapists may experience as a strength or weakness when compared to others in the field.

The normal curve, as in Figure I.1, suggests that very few therapists will rate very high or very low in the above indexes of success. The greatest number of therapists will be in the average range of abilities. Any of the preceding variables could be used in place of the missing words in the following sentences.

Using the variable of (any of the above), the normal curve would suggest that very few therapists will either have a very high or low amount of _____, but most therapists experience a moderate (average) amount of _____. If a therapist views _____ as an important measure of success, then appropriate emphasis, training, and experiences in _____ would be helpful in attaining a desired level of success.

Example using the concept of "clients' goals met"

Using the variable of clients' goals met, the normal curve would suggest that very few therapists will either have a very high or low amount of clients' goals met, but most therapists experience a moderate (average) amount of clients' goals met. If a therapist views clients' goals met as an important measure of success, then appropriate emphasis, training and experiences in clients' goals met would be helpful in attaining a desired level of success.

ENJOYING THE PRICE OF SUCCESS

Success in any field demands a price. Those who sit back and wait for opportunities will do well at times, but in a random manner. Success is not attained by stumbling upon random opportunities, but, rather, by purposely making or opening up opportunities. Successful people do not live in the shadows or achievements of others, but set their own personal and professional goals. They pay a price for operating outside of their safety net.

Many mental health professionals prefer feeling safe in their career paths. The comfort of working for others, a steady paycheck, regular working hours, health insurance, and not having to make major financial and administrative decisions in a clinic can be quite appealing. For many therapists, a safe career path defines success, while for others, success requires leaving their safety net. The following example demonstrates how a safety net, for some people, satisfies some needs, but not all.

Straying from one's safety net clearly requires risk taking. This text describes several areas of potential risk faced by therapists seeking success in their field. Risks can be viewed either as insurmountable barriers or as potential areas for growth. A successful person must first realize that there will be many failures and even more obstacles to hamper his or her efforts for success. Some of these obstacles include competitors, fellow workers, financial

---

Example of One Therapist's View of Success

I was recently referred to conduct a psychological evaluation at a large institution. Prior to seeing the client, I held a conversation with an employee who had been working there for 20 years as a therapist. The conversation went something like this:

Writer: How long have you worked here?

Employee: I've been here over 20 years.

W: Wow, that's great! You must really love your job to be here that long.

E: No, I can't stand working here, but I get a pension in 5 more years, and the insurance benefits are great. I'm just putting in my time. I've been here long enough that they won't fire me, so I just do what I have to do. Maybe when I get my pension I'll try private practice or teach or something.

---

restraints, past failures, fear of failure, fear of success, time, lack of training or experience, improper training, fear of risk taking, feeling comfortable with the status quo, lack of energy, low motivation, too many irons in the fire, family pressures, and the list goes on. Each item on this list is very real and should not be taken lightly.

There are careless risk takers and calculated risk takers. Sometimes the price of a risk is too high compared to the potential gain. Risk always involves uncertainty. There are no guarantees. Thus, all risks should be calculated risks. Each decision should be carefully weighed considering the consequences of failure. For example, when making a decision about leaving a steady job to start a private practice, consideration of all benefits, risks, and alternative courses of action is necessary. In this case, many people starting a private practice will remain in their current position as their new practice develops. It is ethical to inform one's employer of this action in order to avoid a conflict of interests. Some bridges should not be burned. Careless risk takers might appear to be enthusiastic and goal oriented, but they do not consider the potential costs and drawbacks of a course of action before they dive into a new venture. In such cases the outcome is usually eventual failure and often depression. Informative risk taking is the key.

SUCCESS IS NOT WHAT YOU DO; IT IS WHAT YOU ARE

Some of the reasons for aspiring to be successful include increased independence, self-esteem, productivity, recognition in the field, income, personal growth, business acumen, and therapeutic effectiveness. Success is not what you do, but what you are. Although this book will discuss a number of how-to strategies for growing and managing a clinic, without an inner drive to succeed they are no more than additional irons in the fire. A clinic's or a therapist's success is not determined by the number of services provided, but by the quality of those services.

Therapists who continually strive to do their best in several areas will enjoy the benefits of their work. They do not give up when a new plan doesn't work, but, rather, they view the experience as educational and do better next time. They see the whole picture, rather than where they are at the moment. When they work on a job with many negative aspects, they do not complain, but benefit from the experience and are part of the solution.

Example of Which Students Seem to do Well in the Mental Health Field

Besides working in private practices, I have taught graduate and undergraduate psychology students since the mid-1980s and have noticed some distinct features of students who eventually do well in the field, compared to those who do not. Students who do not fare well tend to be eager to complain (especially behind the teacher's back), do not finish assignments on time, regularly ask for time extensions on assignments, minimally read their textbook, and do not interact in class. Studying mental health treatment does not seem to excite them. Successful students respond in an opposite manner. They are eager to learn because becoming a therapist is their life's ambition.

Such behaviors seem to correspond to professional success. Student behaviors such as late homework, complaining, not keeping up, and lack of interaction are akin to such areas as tardiness in writing reports, negativity, not keeping up with professional advancements, and not interacting with other professionals. Each of these behaviors is a matter of choice and habit, rather than unchangeable characteristics. One is never challenged when taking the easy road. Growth is painful, but you grow!

With adequate motivation, direction, training, and supervision, a therapist can be quite successful in the mental health field. Those desiring to go into clinic management have a good start, but there are additional skills to learn. The following chapters provide training in a number of these skills.

1

Basic Mental Health Care Management Principles

This chapter is intended to provide an overview of management responsibilities, whereas the later chapters provide specific techniques and identify the skills needed to provide effective management.

Business management principles in mental health care are no different than other businesses; there are vendors and there are consumers. Some clinics prosper, while others remain stagnant or go out of business. Some develop a positive reputation, while others do not. Although there are no guarantees, there are sound business practices that increase one's chance of success.

A keen knowledge of both the consumer and the vendor must be mastered to remain competitive. A typical midsize mental health clinic does not hire a business manager, due to financial restraints. This duty usually falls upon others who also have clinical duties. Even if a business-oriented manager is hired, there are several mental health clinical skills associated with the position in which clinical training and experience are needed.

Mental health care is becoming more of a business in which professional peers and referral sources are also competitors (in a business sense). The price of trying to compete for business increases the cost of staying in business and decreases the time available to treat clients. Without it, however, a clinic can lose its competitive edge. Plus, without appropriate business skills, the quality of services can decline due to the effects of poor management. Thus, any mental health service provider who has any inkling of becoming a clinical supervisor, director, or manager should receive management training either formally or informally.

With the rise of competition for mental health consumers, one cannot avoid the decision whether to be competitive. Ignoring competition only leads to decreased business. Imagine two retail stores, located on the same block, who sell similar products. Store A's philosophy is, "It has always been our policy to make a 40 percent profit and to only sell articles that are made in this state. That's the way we've always done it, and that's the way we'll always do it." Store B's philosophy is, "If we want to grow and be competitive we will make a profit of 35 percent and we will advertise letting everyone know that our customers will have a greater variety of choices and we sell for less." It is likely that Store B will make a little less money per sale, and have more advertising costs, but the volume of business will more than make up for it. Store A might keep its loyal customer base due to its exclusive product line, but could also go out of business due to not keeping up with the market. Likewise, clinics must know their competition and make ongoing decisions based on market changes.

HOW DO CLINICS BECOME COMPETITIVE?

The answer is as simple or complicated as monitoring prices and services. Consumers want the best quality product for the least possible price. Maintaining this balance maintains one's competitive edge. Clinics that charge too low a price, or pay excessive salaries or commissions, will likely go out of business in a relatively brief period of time. Likewise, if they provide the utmost in high-quality services, their expenses could be quite high. For example, in today's professional sports the ratio of quality to price has made it very difficult for team owners. The team's consumers (those who attend the games and purchase team products) want the team to sign the best players—with contracts in the multimillion dollar range—but they do not want to pay a high price for tickets. A team with mediocre players might have low-price tickets, but there might not be much demand (low ticket sales) due to a losing season. A delicate balance of what can be afforded versus what can be charged is difficult. In mental health, a clinic does not receive more money from third-party payers for their high-end players (seasoned therapists), although there is typically a rate difference between masters and doctoral level therapists. But, seasoned clinicians typically demand a higher salary, and rightfully deserve it. Thus, when a clinic cannot afford high-salaried employees, it must increase its quality of care by other means (see Chapter 2, Customer Service).

Studebaker automobile dealers are no longer in business as Studebaker dealers. They either want out of business or changed brands. Mental health clinics that hold on to outmoded services and business practices must either expand the services they provide or face a downward spiral in business. Mental health consumers are not different from consumers for other businesses. I frequently receive phone calls from prospective clients asking questions such as the prices of services, time frames, location, and payment options. Such questions are remarkably similar to those asked in retail situations. Thus, an effective manager monitors client questions posed to the receptionist—and any others who deal with the consumers—to help the clinic become more desirable or competitive in those areas. This is comparable to a retail store that does not sell a certain product, but due to numerous client requests begins stocking the product, and thus makes a profit. This is not to suggest immediately hiring therapists who specialize in fad treatments or therapies, but does suggest keeping up with market needs for business survival.

At this point in time, the typical model of mental health care management training for students is not through academic training, but through observation of the management practices where they receive their clinical training. The quality of this experience is proportionate to the managerial abilities of their supervisor. If the supervisor is ill-trained or not business oriented, the supervisee will perpetuate the incompetence. If they happen to learn from a business-oriented model, they might do quite well, if they incorporate what they learned.

A small mental health private practice usually has about three to five employees, including one administrative person and a few therapists. The business portion of the practice involves answering the phone, setting up appointments, paying bills, and collecting fees. Many clinics can sustain themselves at this level, but they may or may not grow to be a competitive force.

The larger the clinic, the more a business-like model is needed. Larger clinics have a better chance of receiving the more lucrative contracts. However, due to the increased number of services available, these contract providers impose additional requirements on the clinic to protect their clients and investment. For example, some larger contracts require clinic accreditation or medical personnel on staff. The accrediting process involves disclosure of some very specific policies and procedures. Thus, a larger clinic is much more accountable to outside sources than a small private practice. Terms such as *policies and procedures handbooks, business plans, fiscal management,* and *utilization review committees* are likely foreign to a small clinic, but are part of the everyday lingo in larger clinics.

THREE NECESSARY SKILLS FOR EFFECTIVE CLINIC MANAGEMENT

Historically, we have assumed that the same skills employed in counseling are sufficient for management. Indeed, some of these skills transfer. For example, much of a therapist's training involves people skills, crisis management, and assertiveness. But, are these skills sufficient to manage a clinic? Several additional, specific managerial skills are needed, which are not part of clinical training. Just as a good business manager without clinical training may not be effective in a clinical setting, a good clinician may be unprepared for managerial duties without appropriate training.

Some therapists easily transition into management, while others are ineffective, no matter how effective they may be as a therapist. Clearly, the skills of therapy are necessary, but not sufficient, for management skills. The combination of at least three global skills is necessary for the therapist/manager. These include therapeutic skills, administrative skills, and relational skills. Clinical skills are needed to understand the vision of the clinic, supervise therapists, review charts, hire appropriate clinical staff, and evaluate the services of the clinic. Administrative skills are needed to organize, plan, manage, budget, market, and make the business and personnel decisions necessary for the clinic to function. Relational skills are extremely important to maintain a cohesive group, communicate, and lead a group of divergent people. Any two of these skills is not sufficient without the third.

The model of managerial training, just as in clinical skills, requires training, supervision, and experience. Many a therapist's financial downfall has been to purchase an established clinic before acquiring any managerial experience.

Mental health care providers face the additional challenge of not wanting to appear to the public as a competitive business. They

---

Example of a Good Therapist, but Poor Manager

A small, but thriving, practice had a healthy referral base, provided an array of services, and maintained a healthy income for its owner and employees. The owner decided to sell the practice due to other opportunities. A therapist with excellent clinical skills, but no significant business experience, purchased the practice.

After several months in business the new owner began to see a decline in business and complained to the seller that the clinic was not profitable, suggesting that the seller was misleading in the transaction. The seller then asked the buyer what was being done to maintain and increase business. The new owner's response clearly described the reason for the declines. The response was that no advertising was going out because the level of business when the business was sold was plenty of work.

Lesson: In most mental health clinics, the sources of referrals and revenue change over time. A referral source may be strong for several years, but may stop suddenly because of changes in personnel or other reasons. Often, when personnel change at a referral source, they send their referrals to those they know in the field, rather than the status quo. Thus, when one of your referral sources changes personnel, be sure to immediately develop a relationship. They may quickly begin referring to their previous contacts. The process of seeking new referrals should continue even when business is brisk.

Losing referral sources is not uncommon and should be expected. Thus, marketing strategies must be ongoing, because referral sources are not permanent. This clinic did not replace lost referral sources, thus there was a drop in business.

do not have the luxury of certain retail stores who make advertising claims such as, "We slash the competitor's prices." No one thinks anything about these claims other than as a part of a marketing scheme for a retail business. Or, when an advertising slogan such as "You'd be crazy not to shop here" is heard, people might even think it's humorous. However, if a mental health clinic made such claims, it would likely be viewed as money-grubbing, tacky, providing low-quality services, and clearly not very professional. A high standard is clearly required in the marketing of mental health services.

Not every business decision in mental health treatment can be competitive or have a profit motive. For example, providing a certain percentage of free or low-cost services for the disadvantaged is not only an ethical practice, but it is also expected. Such a practice also allows clients, the public, and clinicians to realize the compassionate, altruistic side of the business, and reinforces the public's typically high perception of mental health therapists. The concept of a competitive clinic, to some therapists, might seem like a paradox.

As mentioned previously, mental health clinic management involves three primary skills, clinical management, and business management. Deficits in any of these areas shortchanges the clinic. The remainder of this book provides training in these areas, whereas this chapter discusses general principles. The remaining chapters also provide specific examples of needed managerial clinical and business skills.

For the sake of communication the title of the person who manages the clinic will be referred to in this text as the clinic director/manager. In very large clinics, these might be two separate positions.

Therapeutic Skills

A mental health clinic director/manager is typically a seasoned therapist experienced in therapy, mental health crises, documentation, upgrading professional credentials, professional presentations, staff training, dealing with ethical issues, the ups and downs of being a therapist, and both supervising and being supervised. Although this person may have little initial experience in managing the administrative aspects of a clinic, there should be a solid track record of complying with both clinical and administrative procedures required by the clinic and the mental health field.

A therapist who cuts corners, provides poor documentation, constantly complains and degrades the clinic, or is passive-aggressive is not a good candidate for management. This does not suggest that a manager must be a "yes-person," but it does mean that the person should not be antiauthoritarian or a clinic policy-breaker. A therapist who has a history of poor compliance with administrative procedures likely does not understand the importance of those procedures and will not suddenly become an administrative role model. Thus, if a potential clinic manager is being promoted from out of the ranks, this person, besides being a seasoned therapist, should have a strong history of following the rules that he or she will later oversee.

Administrative Skills

Clinical Supervision

A clinical director/manager has several clinical management duties. Whether these duties are accomplished through various committees, clinical administrative staff (mid-management), or directly by the clinic director/manager, this person is ultimately responsible for the quality of clinical care at the clinic. Simply assigning senior therapists the task of supervising novice therapists is not sufficient. Minimally, the senior therapists should report to the director/manager for supervision and case management. In smaller clinics the clinic director might provide the clinical supervision.

Case management is clearly more than simply signing off cases. It also provides an opportunity for therapists to grow professionally by discussing their viewpoint and listening to different perspectives about their client's concerns. The supervisor brings additional insight and challenges through extensive experience. Case management duties help the manager/clinic director to learn the strengths and weakness of the clinic's therapists, and provide direction to aid in clinic and client growth. In case management I ask the supervisee to respond to the following types of questions.

Examples of Case Review Questions in Clinical Supervision

1. What is the reason for the referral?

2. What is the client's presenting problem?

3. What are the symptoms leading to the diagnosis? How do they fit the *Diagnostic and Statistical Manual* criteria?

4. How did you rule out (e.g., suicide, chemical dependency, personality disorders, [depending on the case])?

5. What are the resulting impairments?

6. What are the client's strengths, needs, abilities, and preferences (SNAPS)?

7. Are services medically necessary? Why? Why not?

8. How does the treatment plan address these impairments in an objective, measurable manner?

9. Are there any concerns with suicide/homicide?

10. Are there any Chemical Dependence issues?

11. What are the estimated number of sessions?

12. What therapeutic school of thought or techniques do you plan on using? Why?

13. Are any referrals necessary?

14. Should anyone else be involved in the treatment?

15. How effective is the current treatment? How? Why?

16. What changes are needed to best suit the client's needs?

17. What progress has taken place?

18. What are the discharge and aftercare plans?

19. What struggles have you experienced in this case?

20. Are there any ethical issues that need to be addressed?

21. What would you do differently?

22. What have you learned from this case?

Now, provide clinical insight into the case and continue to discuss.

Chart Review

Reviewing charts is different from clinical supervision. It is typically called utilization review (UR) by third parties, involving reviewing the documentation in the charts of therapists at the clinic. Once again, the larger the clinic, the higher the chance that this process will be performed by a UR committee, directed by the clinic director/manager.

Reviewing charts is not necessarily a difficult process—the skill is in the knowledge of what to review, providing accurate feedback, and teaching specific skills to therapists to increase the quality of their work. Some of the main responsibilities of the clinic director/manager are to protect the clinic from unethical practices, provide medically necessary services, be accountable for clinical procedures, meet accreditation standards, and any other actions that could occur under his or her direction. Each of these actions is designed to ultimately fit the client's best interest. Thus, this person must be an expert in clinical accountability standards.

Duties, such as keeping up with changes, staff training, and a careful review of charts, are part of the job description. A clinic director/manager without these skills leaves the clinic vulnerable to consequences such as substandard services to clients, an unsuccessful audit, and possible payback of funds collected.

Perhaps one of the biggest issues therapists have is record keeping. They may have been taught a different system, or no system, at the various clinics where they previously worked. Very few were taught such skills in graduate school. Thus, the clinic director/manager is a supervisor, a teacher, and a mentor, and is responsible for the results of those who are supervised.

Staff Development

The clinic director/manager is responsible for staff training, credentialing, and development. Moderate and large size clinics routinely conduct staff training to help develop new competencies in their therapists. It is not uncommon to hold monthly staff meetings in which a portion of the meeting involves staff training. Topics such as therapeutic techniques, crisis management, safety procedures,

Example of How a Clinic Director / Manager Should Be an Example to Others

I once worked at a clinic where the clinic director was a fine therapist and a natural leader. As part of his managerial style, he regularly admonished therapists to provide proper documentation because the clinic held a very lucrative contract in which audits took place about every 2 years. After each audit the clinic typically was required to pay back several thousand dollars due to the lack of documentation. The director relied on committees to review charts, rather than become involved, but the committee was not allowed to review the clinic director's charts. When the director's charts were audited, the auditors were quite amazed that few notes were kept at all, thus much of the payback to the insurance company was due to the poor documentation of the director.

Lesson: Be sure that the clinic director/manager is more than just aware that accountability standards exist. Be sure that this person, or yourself, is experienced and expert in utilization procedures to the point it is not a burdensome task, but rather a necessary part of the job, leading to better client care and accountability.

compliance guidelines, and much more are covered. Either outside speakers or clinicians at the clinic provide the training.

Established clinics have credentialing guidelines. That is, there are established policies and procedures used to determine which therapeutic procedures may be practiced by each therapist. Typically the guidelines are based on training, experience, and supervision. New therapists must be credentialed within the clinic for each procedure and client demographic (e.g., age group, type of therapy, level of impairment, diagnosis categories). Established therapists present evidence of current training, experience, and supervision to add to their credentials. Once again, the credentialing process might be conducted by the clinic director/manager or via a committee, with final approval by the clinic director/manager.

Some clinics pay for all or part of continuing educational experiences for therapists and administrative staff. Typically, the clinic director/manager or an assigned administrative staff member keeps a record of staff training and continuing education of clinical staff. This information is part of what is reviewed by accreditation agencies and is part of the therapist's annual review by the clinic.

Hiring

Just like any other business, a mental health clinic must have business partners, employees, or independent contractors to provide services. Hiring the right employees is both a science and an art. That is, both objective and subjective information must be integrated. Some applicants look great on paper, but in person they leave a negative impression. Others say very little during the interview, leaving a vague impression, but turn out to be excellent listeners in therapy.

Employees can either make or break an institution. Therefore, the hiring process must be patient, carefully planned, and thorough. Applicants should be interviewed by a few departments within the clinic (e.g., other therapists, management, administrative staff). Previous employment, education, professional references, a criminal background check, and inquiries to their licensing board are a must. Some employers conduct a credit bureau check. Be sure to obtain written permission to conduct these inquiries.

A clinic in immediate need of new therapists must not be too hasty to hire people to fill vacancies. It is better to be a little short of help for a few weeks than hastily hire people who might not be beneficial to the clinic over the long run. It is likely better for clients to be referred elsewhere, or miss a few sessions, than see an inappropriate therapist who wasn't adequately screened.

The final step culminates with the clinic director/manager making a decision and an employment offer. Oftentimes, negotiating begins at this stage. Rarely hire a therapist at a significantly higher pay rate than established therapists at the clinic. Some therapists with higher financial needs will try to negotiate a fairly high salary or commission rate. As a clinic director/manager you will have to make business decisions regarding the feasibility of paying someone a high rate of pay. If the income to the clinic justifies his or her pay, it is generally not an issue. But, if their services pay no more than other therapists, it may not be fiscally responsible to hire this person. Also, some therapists are paid a higher salary or commission based on additional duties beyond conducting therapy (e.g., supervising, case management, administrative duties).

Depending on the size and resources of the clinic the clinic

Example of Budgeting Concerns

In the several years I have worked in clinic management I have come to the realization that commission rates paid to therapists over 60–65 percent lead to little or no profit to the clinic, when considering expenses. That is, the clinic can usually meet expenses paying at these rates, but when hard times come, there is little or no reserve to take care of these issues. Commission rates of about 50–55 percent (without other benefits) provide a fair balance to both the therapist and the clinic. Lower commission rates (without other benefits) typically result in a fairly low income to the therapist and higher turnover. Oftentimes, clinics that pay low commissions or salaries tend to hire novice therapists who are there to get their first job experience.

---

director/manager may also be responsible for scheduling, office hours, office assignments, approving vacation times, advertising, purchases, office leases, referrals, matching intakes to therapists, marketing, budgeting, and a host of other responsibilities if there is not an administrator with such duties.

Relational Skills

Without appropriate relational skills the most effective therapist manager is not able to lead, listen, develop trust, or communicate very well. Having sound clinical skills does not guarantee having good relational skills. This aspect of the job involves dealing with people individually and in groups. They must represent the clinic to clients, therapists, third party payers, accrediting agencies, vendors, referral sources, and several others. The clinic director/manager is typically a direct representation of the clinic.

MANAGEMENT STYLES

Although there are several management styles, the fit between the manager and those being managed is crucial for effective leadership. For example, an authoritarian manager typically encounters many problems with insubordination and discontented employees in a mental health clinic. Therapists typically desire democratic leadership. Leadership in a mental health facility takes a "walking on eggshells" approach when balancing being competitive in the business world and people-oriented in the clinician world. Many therapists simply will not view the clinic as a business entity, as if the clinic will take care of itself if quality services are provided. This naive perspective is perhaps one of the greatest reasons many private practices go out of business in a relatively short period of time.

Texts in leadership skills describe a number of leadership styles. However, this text does not provide such descriptions, because they are much more descriptive in focus, while this text is more prescriptive. That is, not much is included in this text describing clinic management, as it favors providing training on how and what to manage.

For therapists who begin a solo practice that eventually grows to the level of hiring a few therapists, management skills develop

---

Example of Employee Turnover Due to Change in Management

The manager's style is often reflected in the staff of a clinic. I once purchased a clinic from a therapist who had a very different management style than mine. Over the first several months of ownership, clinic morale seemed quite low. Many of the therapists made comparisons between the previous owner and me, stating that things used to be better with the previous owner. Over time a number of the dissatisfied clinicians left the clinic on their own volition (they weren't fired) and were replaced.

It seemed that the bulk of the clinicians that remained and the new clinicians were more in sync with my style of leadership. After the transition took place, clinic morale increased. When I eventually sold the clinic, the same process took place. A different group of people rose to leadership.

Today the clinic still exists, two owners later, with many changes in the clinical staff that fit the current owner's style of leadership. The clinic is doing quite well. None of these staff changes were planned, but the fit between the leadership and staff took place due to leadership needs being fulfilled by some and unfulfilled by others.

Administrative Differences in Managing a
Solo Practice versus a Larger Practice

Solo Practice	Larger Practice
Counseling a full client load	Decreased client load
Obtaining/maintaining a few third party contracts	Obtaining/maintaining several third party contracts
Making policies and procedures as necessary	Producing manuals for policies and procedures that comply with standards from multiple sources
Legally responsible for only your actions	Possible legal responsibility for therapists who work for you
Making all decisions	Regular committee meetings
Few or no staff to manage	Increasing staff with different opinions, backgrounds, availabilities, skills, and so forth
No need for accreditation	To expand business possibilities and reputation, adherence to multiple requirements
No staff issues to manage	Potential staff conflicts, which can lead to disruption in the clinic
More control of working hours	Less freedom in working hours
Payroll is only to you	Must meet payroll, even in lean months
Narrow scope of services	Wide range of services
Potential isolation	Collegiality
Multiple duties	Shared duties

over time. The most difficult aspect of growing into management is attaining the level of business, legal, and management skill needed for the business to grow. The same business principles used to start a solo practice are remarkably different from those used to manage a large clinic.

MAINTAINING A HEALTHY CLINIC
WORK ENVIRONMENT

Clinic management is not a simple task, especially in a large clinic. Office dynamics and politics, such as power struggles, personality clashes, jealousies, dishonesty, employee theft, insubordination, and sycophantic behaviors are not uncommon in some settings. Office struggles will take place in any organization, but when they escalate, it may be indicative of other concerns or disruptions in the clinic. A wise clinic director/manager does not wait for problems to escalate to a crisis level before they are handled, but rather, monitors the pulse of the clinic through nonverbal or indirect indexes of such concerns. The clinic director/manager is not simply the person in the corner office who runs meetings, but rather, the bridge between the clinical and the business side of the clinic.

An effective clinic manager strives to promote a healthy office environment. Unfortunately, in the practice of mental health there can be strife or divisions within a clinic, such as clinical versus nonclinical staff or divisions within a department. A team approach in which cooperative efforts are rewarded can go a long way in promoting unity. Rewarding positive behaviors, rather than waiting to reprimand negative behaviors, is much more effective in achieving a positive office environment. When clinicians and staff members experience a sense of teamwork, unity, and camaraderie, the work environment becomes like a second family to its workers. This positive atmosphere among the staff is felt by the clients. A giving leadership leads to a giving staff. This point cannot be overemphasized.

Unity within a clinic begins at the top tier of management. Fractions, open disagreements, and side-taking that lead to division have no place in effective clinic management. Disruptions that could lead to a perception of interpersonal stress between managers always have an ill effect on morale. Obviously, disagreements will take place, but they should not interfere with morale or the mission of the clinic. Without some dissonance there is no growth; therefore, seek diversity, but do not let it get out of control.

Example of a Manager versus Owner Relationship Breakdown in a Clinic

I have seen far too many clinics begin due to a breakup at another clinic. Many great clinics are no longer in existence because management did not learn how to work together. Perhaps some therapists who go into management are so used to being the authority (in clinical settings) that they are not used to being a team player. Some treat the clinic as if they own it.

Very early in my career I applied to a fairly large mental health center whose director was not the owner or the founder of the clinic, but was partially responsible for the clinic's success. He received a hefty salary, but not as much profit as the owner, who was not on-site. As the clinic grew that clinic director became more vocal regarding his dislike for the owner. Plus, a number of statements were made that he should receive a larger piece of the pie.

I applied for a position at this clinic not knowing about the problems with the disgruntled management. During my interview everyone seemed fairly cordial and the job seemed promising. On Monday I came to work for my clinical orientation. To my surprise, one secretary and I were the only people there! All of the offices were emptied out. I phoned the owner, who knew nothing about why everyone had abruptly left.

It turned out that for several months the clinic director had been planning with every employee, except the secretary, to start a new clinic. They told all of the clients about their new location. Insurance and managed care companies provided the new clinic with appropriate contracts. They even became a licensed facility with the state. This all took place without the owner's knowledge.

On the weekend prior to leaving, most of the staff went to the clinic and copied client files to bring to their new clinic. They even used the clinic's copy machine! The secretary (having a history of loyalty to the owner) came to work knowing nothing about the other employees leaving. The owner had no idea that any problems even existed. In fact, in a staff meeting one week before, the clinic director told the owner everything was going fine. The clinical and administrative staff were simply gone. With no other staff available, the clinic closed down and I had no job.

Lesson: Management and ownership must communicate and share more than the transfer of money. Misunderstandings, communication problems, and resentment can lead to the downfall of a clinic.

PROMOTING A SENSE OF FAIRNESS

Many managerial concerns stem from individual staff members believing that they are working harder than others; thus, they deserve
more compensation, favorable treatment, or attention. This belief
may also lead to disunity among staff and a number of disgruntled
employees. Such problems often stem from vague or changing job
descriptions.

Indeed, a workload seems unfair when others around you are
doing less and being paid the same. In a mental health clinic, however, few people have the same job description; thus, different duties
are expected from different people. For example, if one employee
answers the phone 70 percent of the time and another person answers it 30 percent of the time, the first employee could feel cheated,
unless there is a job description that demarcates the specific duties
for each position. Make all efforts to assure that employees are not
given too many or too few duties. Periodically conduct a job analysis
with the end result of placing employees on a level playing field.
However, do not stifle employees' abilities and room for growth by
limiting them to their job descriptions.

There should be clearly spelled out job descriptions, expectations, salary levels, benefits, and any information associated with
the position. Rather than hiring special employees provide equal
opportunities for all employees. Promotions should come by merit
and qualifications. Objectively document specific reasons for pro-
moting/demoting or increasing/decreasing the salary levels of employees. Promote a work environment where the employees are
there primarily for the job satisfaction, not only the pay.

A manager whose attitude reflects being part of a team is more
likely to develop a smoothly working team if this is his or her true intention. It is difficult to feign truly caring about employees; it must
be genuine. The combination of business skills, coupled with therapeutic and people skills, makes for a great clinic director/manager.

THE KEY TO SUCCESSFUL MENTAL HEALTH CLINIC MANAGEMENT: EMPOWERMENT

One of the least successful management styles in most businesses and mental health is an authoritarian style. Mental health therapists are well educated and clearly able to make important decisions. Their frame of mind is empowerment. Therapists spend much time treating clients by encouraging assertiveness and self-actualization behaviors, thus teaching empowerment. It is also a part of their lives.

Mental health therapists strive for a sense of being, meaning, and purpose. Being told what to do, with little or no say in the matter, does not contribute to vocational satisfaction. Workers want to be a contributing, responsible, and valued part of the organization they represent. A top-heavy balance of power in a clinic results in high turnover of employees.

An effective manager will encourage clinicians to be their very best, take initiative, and be an active part of the workings of the clinic. Their positive attributes are encouraged. Employees with this sense of purpose in the clinic will rise to the challenge of self-fulfillment. Managers who encourage new ideas, creativity, and openly allow employees to empower themselves will have a highly committed staff.

In the business world, competing businesses often sell the same or similar products. One business is more likely to excel when its employees are innovative and free to be creative, rather than just doing their jobs. The ideas for innovations or changes come from all levels of employees. For example, top management may not be aware of minor but consistent customer complaints or delays in customer service, but when all levels of employees are free to experiment and try new procedures (within reason) effective change can take place. There is a risk of failure in experimentation, but without it, nothing changes and others pass you by.

In a mental health clinic all levels of employees can contribute and be creative in their ideas. For example, the receptionist will likely have the best ideas for improved customer relations, because the receptionist is often the first one to hear customer concerns. They have direct contact with the clinic's client base. When the receptionist is treated as an expert in his or her area, and suggestions

---

Example of an Empowered Therapist

A therapist worked at a clinic for several years. He initially started full-time and was a vital part of the clinic. He led a committee, helped in staff trainings, and was vital in starting a children's mental health program. His helpful suggestions and leadership were appreciated. He felt much self-fulfillment working at the clinic.

After about 6 years a new clinic director with a very different management style was hired. The new clinic director did not like therapists making clinic decisions. All new ideas had to go through the director. The therapist's input and clinic participation soon waned. He remained working at the clinic part-time, but also took a job at another clinic. Eventually, he became a complainer and often talked about the way things used to be.

The clinic director remained at the clinic for about 5 years. The therapist remained working one day per week and was not involved in any committees, staff trainings, or other nonclinical matters. A new clinic director was hired with a managerial style similar to the first clinic director. After about 6 months the therapist, once again, became involved in more aspects of the clinic. His ideas were valued and he once again became a role model of leadership and innovation. Eventually, he returned to full-time work as a very satisfied therapist, regularly contributing to the well-being of the clinic.

Lesson: Leadership that allows workers to empower themselves through creativity, innovation, and working to their potential can find itself managing a very dynamic clinic with satisfied employees.

---

and innovations are given a chance, the receptionist becomes part of the leadership of the clinic and is motivated to be more helpful. The manager who views the receptionist as an underling or subordinate, and does not provide the receptionist with opportunities to grow and find self-fulfillment in the clinic, will have a stagnant office staff with little or no job satisfaction. Staff turnover not only lowers morale, but is also very expensive.

Caution When Empowering Employees

The term *empowering* employees is actually not empowerment, but rather, a misnomer. That is, if the clinic leadership allows or permits employees to have more job role flexibility, what actually takes place is continued oversight of more duties. Empowerment must also include leadership yielding some power as employees take on leadership roles based on initiative, not mandate. Thus, for some managers, empowerment can be viewed as threatening.

Empowerment can be quite difficult in mental health management. For example, clinics who tend to receive higher ratings from accreditation sources and obtain more contracts often have very detailed policies and procedures, which are designed to impress the agencies. When employees become creative and bypass policies, it could lead to reprimands. If a manger is authoritarian, it is possible that the least creative employees could receive promotions due to their compliance. However, too much conformity leads to becoming stagnant. If there are too many layers of management in a clinic, the possibility of an idea being squelched increases with each layer if only the top level makes the final decisions. A typical hierarchical model can be the worst enemy of innovation and progress.

There must be a balance between conformity and creativity in a clinic. I suggest that management regularly encourage creativity in the form of ideas and discussions at staff meetings, where all employees have an equal say in discussions. Better listening leads to better ideas. A pilot project can be considered when an idea seems potentially helpful. Reinforce the creator of the idea and give the idea a chance. If it proves helpful, work it into your policies and procedures. The policies and procedures manual is important, but it is also revisable. All aspects of the clinic are dynamic rather than static.

If every new idea is immediately incorporated into clinic policy, chaos would prevail, but if every new idea is discussed, given a chance to be studied and revised or improved through group action, some of these ideas could be a catalyst for change and an encouragement to others to innovate.

Effective management creates an environment where employees have the freedom to grow, make suggestions without fear of reprisal, take risks that are within reason, and feel as if they are part of the organism of the organization A well-managed organization views the organization as compared to a human body, in which each body part is necessary. That is, the hands, head, heart, and

Example of Management Listening to Employees'
Concerns Leading to Improvements

A clinic had a policy that therapists must collect deductibles and co-payments from clients. The collection rate was fairly poor. A number of therapists complained that it was not their job to collect money, noting that it was personally uncomfortable. Management replied that a therapist collecting the co-payments was therapeutic by helping clients be responsible. Therapists felt pressured and further described collecting fees as adversely affecting the counseling relationship. They didn't know what to do when clients stated that they had no money with them, because it was the clinic's policy to not render services unless the co-payment was met. It would be very difficult to ask a client to leave at the beginning of a session.

In a staff meeting a group of therapists brought up a discussion about their concerns, and further added a suggestion to consider a clinic policy that required clients to make their co-payments and deductibles at the front desk with the receptionist (just like at a medical clinic). Management listened and agreed to give it a try.

For the next few weeks clients were informed of an upcoming policy to make their payments up front before seeing their therapist. Plus, just like in a medical office, this amount must be paid prior to receiving services. Due to the ample warning of the policy change, clients were very compliant with the new procedure.

After an analysis of the percentages and amounts of co-payments and deductibles received, the clinic found that they were taking in a significantly higher amount of money with the same number of clients.

feet each have a function, and the body would not function to its full potential without all of its parts. At times the feet shine, when the organization must move quickly, but at other times the heart is in the forefront, when its caring nature is needed. At other times the hands are needed, when work is to be done. During the course of everyday matters, each member coordinates with each other as the body, not various factions. The head is held up by the rest of the body, but helps organize its efforts. It functions best when the power and energy is distributed to the body in a sufficient amount that it functions at its full potential, not just where one member dictates.

People are not creative when they feel boxed in, ruled, or put down. Nor do they become creative when they are mandated to be creative. It comes from having the freedom to create. Creativity, not being told what to do in all matters, leads to reaching potential.

BALANCING MANDATES AND CREATIVITY

Therapists function best by providing treatment within the realm of their education, beliefs, experiences, and worldview. Their personality style and interpersonal skills go beyond therapeutic techniques. There is always more to learn, but when they are stifled by rules and requirements in a session, the field suffers. Therapy is both an art and a science. When therapists incorporate their personalities, part of their very being becomes incorporated into treatment.

The supervisor who corrects a therapist's counseling style in areas that are nonessential to basic counseling skills but rather are personal traits that happen to be different from the supervisor, may be in danger of stifling the therapist's creativity. The adage, "major on the majors, and minor on the minors," is especially true. Too often, in management, we major on the minors.

Likewise, in other areas of clinic management, people want to feel like an autonomous part of a larger organism. This is not a contradiction, but rather, it is an excellent formula for growth and organizational unity and strength. One's contributions to the organization help promote a sense of purpose. Staff with this type of drive go beyond their job description because that extra mile is a motivator. Everyone benefits.

When employees portray this attitude, acknowledge them and show appreciation. Let them know that their contributions directly increase the quality of the clinic. Employees treated in this manner will find the balance between following the policies and procedures of the clinic and innovating new ideas to improve the current system.

As managers/clinic directors we want to receive the most each employee has to offer. Knowledge is power. An effective organization invests in increasing its employees' competencies. Staff training, seminars, college courses, workshops, job shadowing, graduated levels of experience, and other means of training should be encouraged and subsidized whenever possible. A company of experts working together is on the winning team.

SUMMARY

Knowledge of business management skills is crucial in the operation of a mental health clinic. The clinic director/manager makes decisions that can make or break a clinic financially and in the quality of services offered. A well-organized manager can build a clinic from a small private practice to a large clinic in a relatively few number of years because most of the competition is not trained in business management.

Without adequate training and business acumen, a well-meaning therapist-become-manager can soon spiral to a financial downfall. Problems, including going out of business without the means to pay off business loans, long-term leases, and business equipment, can lead to years of financial woes. Errors resulting from putting all of one's eggs into the same basket can soon break one's nest egg.

Therapists can make excellent clinic managers. Most of them already have two of the three necessary skills for effective mental health clinic management: therapeutic and relational skills. When they receive adequate training in the third area, administrative skills, they are on the right road to managing a successful clinic.

Too many therapists assume that if they have been successful as a clinician they are qualified to manage a clinic. Some therapists do quite well, but many do not readily make the transition, at the expense of the clinic and, ultimately, the clients.

Managers who must be the person in charge and require that all ideas and decisions go through them will suppress their employees' desire to be creative and self-fulfilled in the workplace. This trait is most often found in insecure managers who must have their way. Most therapists, as well as other professionals, desire a place of employment where they are given the freedom to be innovative, creative, and make decisions that could better their job. Managers who encourage this freedom will develop a cohesive, supportive, and professional staff with few limits in their capabilities.

TEST YOUR KNOWLEDGE

1. Which of the following skills are required for a successful mental health clinic manager or director?

   (a) Therapeutic skills

   (b) Administrative skills

   (c) Relational skills

   (d) All of these

2. What is the source of most mental health clinic manager's or director's managerial training?

   (a) Business college

   (b) Graduate school

   (c) Observations of previous supervisors

   (d) None of these

3. What is meant by *empowering* employees?

   (a) Providing an atmosphere in which employees desire to innovate

   (b) Adding to their duties and responsibilities

   (c) Giving them permission to make more decisions

   (d) Rewarding employees for adhering to company policies

4. Effective managers encourage

   (a) adherence to rules and regulations.

   (b) experimenting with new procedures.

   (c) leadership spread out as people rise to the occasion.

   (d) all of these.

5. What is the main difference in the management of a mental health clinic compared to other businesses?

   (a) A mental health clinic makes less profit

   (b) A mental health clinic is a nonprofit agency

    (c) The public's image

    (d) The wage structure of employees

6. Clinic credentialing of therapists is

    (a) required in all mental health clinics.

    (b) an optional practice.

    (c) is required by licensing agencies.

    (d) not necessary because therapists are professionals.

Answers: 1. d; 2. c; 3. a; 4. d; 5. c; 6. b

2

Customer Service

In real estate the three key words to selling a house are *location, location,* and *location.* Dale Carnegie sales training emphasizes three key words to success in sales: *enthusiasm, enthusiasm,* and *enthusiasm.* The success of a mental health clinic also has three concepts of success, which are *customer service, customer service,* and *customer service.* Without customer service even the greatest clinician has few or no clients. A 4.0 graduate school GPA and a perfect score on the national licensure examination has nothing to do with customer service or success in the field of mental health. Professional tests ask no questions about such matters. Graduate schools rarely mention it. The only test of customer service is akin to the old adage *"the proof is in the pudding."* If you do it well, you will earn positive results.

Customer service is the key to keeping existing clients (from premature termination of services) and receiving referrals from several sources. In any business, the product of good customer service is a satisfied consumer who will return for more services and refers others. Although we are not selling a tangible product in mental health, high-quality customer service is no different from any other business. A mental health clinic does not have a separate customer service department, but is just as concerned about maintaining a positive reputation, obtaining repeat business, and receiving new referrals. Everyone is the customer service department. Customer service in mental health goes far beyond being a competent therapist.

Basic counseling skills such as establishing rapport, empathy, genuineness, positive regard, staying on target, professionalism, and expertise not only lead to effective therapeutic outcomes, they also lead to a relationship of trust and overall positive feelings, not just toward the concept of therapy, but also toward the therapist. That is, being an effective therapist certainly increases customer service. Even in cases in which the therapist has no more than a brief telephone contact or only one consultative session, the behavior toward the client will be remembered and can lead to future referrals.

Customer service begins long before therapy takes place. We are living in an era when customer service is becoming too mechanized and does not have enough personalized attention. Consumers are often surprised when they are treated well. A client's first indirect contact with the therapist is the person (or machine) answering the phone. Clients want to talk with a live, friendly, knowledgeable person who can effectively answer any questions and make a timely appointment. They expect a higher quality of customer service from therapists than other businesses. Voice mail and vague answering services are among the biggest reasons potential clients phone another clinic rather than wait for a callback.

Typically, it can be very difficult emotionally for clients to make an initial therapy appointment. The dissonance they feel between

---

Example of Initial Customer Service

I utilize practicum students in my practice. One of the first elements of their training is customer service. Statements such as, "Treat clients like royalty," "Make them feel welcome here," "Smile when they come in," and "We are the friendly clinic," are highly emphasized. These statements hold true, not only for clients, but for people who accompany them in the waiting room, and others who you come in contact with regarding the clinic.

Lesson: Clients that are treated well rarely complain and are more likely to continue in treatment and to refer others. It is equally important to understand that the purpose of treating clients well is not solely in order to get referrals. However, clients who are treated well will generate referrals. Just as in baseball, the runner cannot get to second base without going to first base. If second base is psychotherapy is any therapeutic advance, then first base might be the client feeling warm, trusting, and welcome at the clinic.

deciding to contact a clinic and making an appointment remains stressful until it is resolved by the closure of finally making an appointment. Thus, when they must wait to hear back from someone to get an appointment, they are likely to phone other clinics until they find one that responds immediately.

FIRST IMPRESSIONS OF THE CLINIC

First impressions are everything in a mental health clinic. If that first impression is an answering machine or voice mail, much business will be lost. If the practice cannot yet afford a receptionist, an answering service can provide this service quite well for a fraction of the cost of a full-time receptionist. An answering service is always better than voice mail or an answering machine. An informed person from the clinic answering the phone is better than an answering service.

When considering all factors, a clinic cannot afford to *not* have a live person answering the phone. The small price of an answering machine translates into the large cost of lost business. The price of a live person answering the phone is not an expense; it is an investment.

Clients want service *now* and they want an appointment as soon as possible. If they cannot speak to someone immediately on the phone, they will usually phone the next clinic on the list. Many answering service companies can offer 24-hour service from a remote location where they answer the phone for a number of companies, thus reducing costs. Typically, the therapist provides the answering service with ample information to answer client questions and even make appointments. Usually, clients do not know they are speaking with someone from an answering service—thus, there are rarely any problems when a high-quality service is used. Most phone answering services, but not all, provide excellent customer service training to their employees. If they did not, they wouldn't remain in business. They are able to answer the phone in the name of your clinic because the telephone number clients call is dedicated to the clinic on their switchboard or computer screen. Some answering services specialize in medical or mental health clinics.

However, at any answering service, one of several persons might answer the phone for the clinic. They do not have the emotional investment in the clinic of an employee. Thus, it is important to carefully screen potential answering services to determine what extent of customer service they provide. Are they simply a place that answers your phone, or an integral part of your clinic? Before contracting with an answering service, ask for the names of a few of their clients. Then, at different times of the day, phone the clinics that have that service answer the phone, and ask several questions about the services they offer. This will give you an idea as to how they might represent your practice.

When a new clinic is formed, and therapists' schedules are not filled, they can rotate answering the phones. When they are with clients, they simply forward the calls to the answering service. Some answering services charge by the week or month, and others charge by the number of calls.

When answering the phone speak with enthusiasm, empathy, and interest. Remember that clients are contacting the clinic due to mental health issues, and some of them will be difficult due to their mental health condition, and because they are hurting emotionally. Their reaction might be to lash out at anyone in their way. However, if they are treated with dignity and respect, most people will put their guard down due to your (or the receptionist's) positive attitude toward them—if it appears to be genuine. They may be accustomed to people retaliating when they verbally aggress. Therefore, do not be defensive or offensive; be supporting. The "turn the other cheek" adage is an excellent customer service tool. I have seen many clients' demeanor shift from screaming, threatening, and abusive to whimpering and apologetic when they are treated with warmth and understanding. Role-play these situations with office personnel.

Clients expect mental health clinics to have a higher standard of customer service than other businesses. They typically view a clinic as a place where the employees have entered the field because they care about other people. They may also assume that employees in a mental health facility are friendly people without mental health issues. If clients do not receive warm treatment or do not receive an immediate response, you might never hear from them again. Psychotherapy is a very competitive business. Much is expected; therefore, mental health customer service training is necessary. Although office personnel are not trained therapists, I have often been surprised how clients will open up to nonclinical personnel due to these presuppositions.

WAITING LISTS

In a mental health field it is common for clinics to have a waiting list. It may even seem prestigious for a clinic to boast that they are so busy or in such high demand that clients must wait an appreciable amount of time to see one of their therapists. Business-wise it is better to have too much business than not enough. However, the client may suffer.

Establish a policy eliminating a waiting list, at least most of the time. Do whatever it takes to see a client within a week of the initial contact. Clients phone you when they are ready. In emergency situations, do not require a wait. Each clinic should have an on-call therapist or make an arrangement with a 24-hour crisis counseling center when you cannot be available to someone who needs services immediately.

When you get too busy and perspective clients must wait longer and longer for an appointment, either hire additional therapists or have referral sources readily available who are able to see the client in a reasonable amount of time. At least be able to give perspective clients a choice to wait until a specific appointment time is available, or accept a referral to another clinic. Or, better yet, offer a choice of clinics.

Therapists who do not set limits, can't say no or who do not consider the potential consequences to the client making him or her wait an extended time for an appointment may end up with long waiting lists. In these cases most clients can be referred to other clinics for services. However, a therapist may be the only one in the area who specializes in a specific subspecialty in which no other area therapists are competent to help clients with specific concerns. In such cases, group therapy is sometimes helpful, when appropriate. Sometimes there are simply too many clients needing a therapist's services. Consider training an intern or a fellow professional

> *Example of Customer Service in Advertising Material*
>
> I have found it very beneficial to include statements in advertising material such as "no waiting lists," or "appointments within one week." Some clinics advertise "same day appointments"—however, it may be difficult to follow through on such statements on busy days. Nevertheless, a client who needs help *now* will be attracted to a clinic that can provide timely services, rather than requiring a wait of up to several days or weeks. Of course, there is the paradox that such practices will lead to more business, and the busier you become, the less time you have available to clients.

willing to learn the specialized skill. But, in the meantime, the situation will be difficult for both the therapist and clients in need of these services.

I have received many new referral sources from various agencies because larger clinics have waiting lists beyond the agency's threshold. Waiting lists can lead to a significant loss of business. It is very difficult to regain a referral source once confidence has been lost.

The belief that the client can wait can lead to a disastrous series of events for the client. They generally phone a clinic during a fairly narrow window of opportunity when they are ready for counseling. This window could easily close if the client must wait too long. All reasonable measures to meet the client's needs should be taken, even if it means a loss of business by making a referral. If your clinic is too busy, have alternatives available for new clients.

THE RECEPTIONIST: THIS PERSON CAN MAKE OR BREAK A CLINIC!

There is an added benefit as a clinic grows and can afford to employ someone to answer the phone, because this same person usually also performs other functions, such as greeting clients, scheduling, filing, and billing. Large clinics have separate employees for each of these functions. However, a clinic with only a few therapists rarely needs more than one clerical or administrative employee.

A key person in any successful clinic or mental health practice is the receptionist, who answers the phone and greets clients. The manner in which the receptionist answers the phone, responds to questions, sets of appointments, and converses with clients directly affects the business operations of the clinic. This person gives clients their first impression of the clinic. The receptionist's value to the clinic can be either disastrous or a godsend. An accumulation of several factors, including tone of voice, quality of answers given,

---

Common Questions Asked by Potential Clients

1. What are your hours?

2. Do you accept _____ insurance?

3. What services do you offer? __individual __family __relational __group __in home

4. Do you have a sliding fee? What is it?

5. Do you have payment plans available?

6. How soon can someone see me?

7. Do you have a psychiatrist?

8. Do you have female and/or male therapists?

9. Does anyone specialize in. . . ? (e.g., Obsessive-Compulsive Disorder, eating disorders, thought disorders, Agoraphobia, Attention Deficit/Hyperactivity Disorder, domestic violence, Bipolar, personality disorders, depression, eating disorders, sexual problems, gender issues, various age groups, evaluations)

10. What education and experience does (name of therapist) have?

11. Can you send me literature about the clinic?

12. Do you have a Web site?

13. Which bus routes can I take to the clinic?

14. How many years have you been in business?

15. How much education does (name of therapist) have?

16. What is the difference between (various types of therapists; e.g., marriage and family, psychologist, social worker, psychiatrist).

professionalism, friendliness, knowledge of the clinic, follow-up skills, and nonverbal behaviors can make or break the growth of a clinic.

Many clients will direct a number of questions to the receptionist and decide if they will make an appointment based on the answers they receive. It is highly recommended to have a list of potential questions, with their respective answers, that the receptionist can study, role-play, and have available for an immediate response.

Make a folder that provides the answers to a variety of client questions. Be sure that anyone answering the phone has ready access to the answers of the previously listed questions, or any other questions that could pertain to the services you offer. Have a vita or list of competencies, education, and experience available for every therapist at the clinic. Encourage staff to role-play clients phoning the clinic and asking questions. Also, encourage them to study the folder so their responses to clients do not seem canned or read.

Consider the Following Two Phone Scenarios

Scenario One

Potential Client: I am looking for counseling. Do you have a female therapist who specializes in anxiety disorders?

Receptionist: Yes, we have several therapists.

PC: Do you have a fairly experienced female therapist who specializes in anxiety disorders?

R: I could have someone call you with that information.

PC: How long does it take to get an appointment with someone?

R: It really varies. I'll have someone phone you.

PC: How do I pay for services?

R: I'll have someone call you back to discuss this.

Scenario Two

Potential Client: I am looking for counseling. Do you have any female therapists who specialize in anxiety disorders?

Receptionist: Yes, we have two experienced female therapists who specialize in anxiety disorders.

PC: Could you tell me a little about them.

R: (Using a prepared sheet with therapist's qualifications, goes over

---

Example of a Great Receptionist

The head receptionist in a large mental health clinic in Troy, Michigan, Kelley Deluge, is well liked by all clients. She always greets them with a welcoming smile and quickly learns their names, establishing immediate rapport. If she is off work, clients ask, "Where's Kelley?" Although she does not have a degree in mental health, the therapeutic process starts with her. She does not discuss clients' mental health concerns with them, but simply treats them as important people—not because it is her job, but because they are important to her. Staff members of this caliber are priceless to a clinic.

---

   specific information that the therapists have supplied about their credentials)

PC: What options are there to pay for services?

R: We accept most insurances and we have a sliding scale fee for those who cannot afford our regular rates.

PC: How long does it take to get an appointment with someone?

R: Both Dr. Troy and Dr. Corral have openings in the next week. Would you like to schedule an appointment at this time?

PC: Yes, what times does Dr. Corral have available next week?

   The second scenario is clearly superior to the first because the receptionist was well informed when asked basic questions. The receptionist appeared to be part of the clinic team, rather than someone who simply answers the phone.

Therapist Information That is Helpful to the Receptionist

The following form provides examples of the types of information a receptionist should refer to when matching therapists to clients. It narrows down the clinic's therapists into specialty areas according to their competencies and preferences. Then, the receptionist can turn to the therapists' information form or vita and provide more specific information if requested. Thus, when a client makes a request for a certain therapist's qualifications, the receptionist or intake coordinator can first turn to the checklist to narrow down the

Example of Competency Sheet to Help Match Clients to Therapists

Therapist

Competencies	1 (M, SW)	2 (F, PS)	3 (F, M&F)	4 (M, PS)	5 (F, M&F)	6 (M, M&F)	7 (F, PC)	8 (M, PC)	9 (M, PS)
Client group									
Children	X			X					X
Adolescents	X		X		X	X		X	X
Adults		X	X		X	X		X	X
Seniors		X	X		X	X	X	X	X
Diagnosis									
ADHD	X			X					
Anxiety		X		X	X		X	X	
Behavioral Disorders	X			X		X			
Crisis Counseling						X	X		
Depression	X	X		X		X	X	X	
Bipolar	X			X		X	X		
Substance Abuse			X						
Developmental Delays	X			X					
Eating Disorders	X								
OCD					X			X	
Panic Attacks					X		X		
Thought Disorders					X			X	
Other _____									

Treatment

Treatment	1	2	3	4	5	6	7	8	9
Individual Counseling	X	X		X	X	X	X	X	
Groups	X		X		X	X	X		
Marriage and Family	X		X	X	X	X		X	
Behavioral	X	X	X						
Cognitive		X	X						
Humanistic/Existential				X		X	X		
Psychodynamic					X			X	
Testing/Evaluations		X		X					X
Other EMDR			X						
Other Personality Disorders						X			
Other _____									

Notes: M = male; F = female; M&F = marriage and family; PC = professional counselor; PS = psychologist; SW = social worker.

possibilities of therapists. Then the specific information about therapists who match the general request can be compared to make a better match.

This system also prevents unnecessary client visits to therapists who do not have the competencies they require. If no one in the clinic suitably fits the client's needs (or request for a specialty area) a referral can be made, saving the client time and preventing the use of unneeded services. Each therapist should have a clinic-approved competency in each of the areas endorsed.

COMPARING THE CUSTOMER SERVICE OF 40 CLINICS

In an informal survey conducted for the purposes of writing this book, 40 mental health clinics of various sizes were contacted by phone and asked several questions regarding their availability and types of services.

Survey Results

This is considered an informal, nonscientific survey. It is limited to a large metropolitan area and its suburbs. A total of 44 practices were phoned during normal business hours. The practices were chosen through *Yellow Page* ads and listings, ranging from basic listings to larger ads. Thus, practices that do not advertise in *The Yellow Pages* had no chance of being surveyed. An equal number of clinics were phoned from the various sizes of ads. All phone calls were made between 10:00 A.M. to 12:00 P.M. and 1:00 P.M. to 4:00 P.M. These times were chosen because they are hours when one might expect a phone to be answered in a business.

Number of clinics contacted	44
Number of clinics not returning phone call	4

Thus, the survey is based on 40 responses.

Clinics directly answering the phone on first attempt — 19 (48%)

Clinics using voice mail or an answering machine — 16 (40%)

Clinics using an answering service — 5 (12%)

Average time to wait for response when a message was left — 3.5 hours

Questions	Responses	
1. How soon can I get an appointment?	95% within a week	5% waiting list
2. Do I have a choice of therapists?	Yes (27, 68%)	No (13, 32%)
3. Is both group and individual counseling available?	Yes (20, 50%)	No (20, 50%)
4. Does the clinic have a Web page?	Yes (12, 30%)	No (28, 70%)
5. Are psychiatric services referrals available?	Yes (23, 58%)	No (17, 42%)
6. Do you accept most insurances?	Yes (34, 85%)	No (6, 15%)
7. Do you have a sliding scale fee schedule?	Yes (11, 27%)	No (29, 73%)
8. Do you have evening/weekend appointments available?	Yes (12, 30%)	No (28, 70%)
9. Are 24-hr emergency services available?	Yes (8, 20%)	No (32, 80%)
10. Is the office located near public transportation?	Yes (24, 60%)	No (16, 40%)
11. How many therapists work there?	Average: 7.3	Range: 1–25
12. How many years has the clinic been in business?	Average: 14.2	Range: 1–30

Points to Ponder

Although this survey is not scientific, it does represent a sample of a large metropolitan area. Almost all of the clinics surveyed have services available within 1 week. One large and one small clinic stated that they have waiting lists of up to a few weeks at a time.

Concerns are noted in that most practices do not have 24-hour emergency services available, such as a therapist on call. However, in their voice mail most provide an outside number to phone, such as 911 or a local crisis center. Large clinics typically have someone on call, so that someone may be paged when the clinic is not open. Some therapists provide clients with their personal phone number, but this is not a common practice, nor do I suggest it.

The number of therapists working at a clinic was proportionate to the size of their *Yellow Pages* ad. There were no solo practices with large ads. Some larger, established clinics had smaller ads, likely due to less need for advertising because of a strong, established reputation.

The main concern is the lack of response during the initial phone call. Less than one half of the clinics surveyed directly answered their phone. Of the five clinics that utilized an answering service, three of those services could only answer a few basic questions about the clinic. When we left a request for a call back from the clinic with an answering service, voice mail, or answering machine the average time for a clinic response was about 3.5 hours. Significant concerns are noted in the four clinics that did not return a phone call.

About one third of the clinics contacted stated there was not a standard fee for services, explaining that the fee depends upon which therapist the client will see. They further noted that different clinicians accept different insurances. These procedures are clearly confusing to the public. Such policies would be unheard of in a medical or dental practice. However, the public is likely not aware that third parties, in mental health insurance, typically credential therapists individually in smaller clinics. It is a common practice in a mental health clinic to have one fee for a master's level clinician and a higher fee for doctoral level clinicians. However, when individual therapists charge different fees for reasons other than their level of licensure, it may appear there is a lack of consistency in the clinic. A wide range of fees is most common when the clinicians are independent contractors, rather than clinic employees. If your clinic has a wide range of fees, disclose this information to consumers. In addition, inform them of the employment status of therapists (i.e., employee, partner, independent contractor).

This delay in response will clearly decrease the number of appointments made. Clinics that can make an immediate appointment provide a much higher level of customer service. A clinic can provide an array of services, but if clients cannot get in touch with the clinic immediately, those clients will find services elsewhere.

FIRST IMPRESSIONS OF THE OFFICE

Even before the client speaks personally to the receptionist the appearance of the building and inside of the office form a clear impression. First impressions such as, "The walls are marked up, the carpet is dirty, the artwork is cheap or inappropriate, no one here is friendly, the offices aren't soundproofed, everything seems so clinical," and so on, will certainly affect the potential client's view of the clinic and thus, the therapist. The office does not have to be exorbitantly decorated, but it should be clean and welcoming. Most mental health clients are looking for a place where they will feel welcomed, not just like another number. They are seeking services because they need help. They do not want to feel ignored or swept aside. Perhaps one of the reasons they seek a therapist's services is because of this type of treatment by others in their lives. The attitudes of all office personnel must be that of care, warmth, and client interest. Periodic staff training in these areas is time well spent.

It may be helpful to furnish the office at a comfortable level concomitant with those who will be seen in the practice. That is, low-income clients who may be used to simple surroundings might feel uncomfortable in a lavish setting, and vice versa. When in doubt, simplicity is the best option.

Now that the client has walked into the clinic and has made an impression of the surroundings, typically the first person he or she comes in contact with is the receptionist. This may or may not be the same person who answered the phone. Client impressions of the clinic become further ingrained by the demeanor of the receptionist. By this point the client is likely ill at ease due to the impending therapy appointment with a stranger in the next few minutes. What is needed is a calm, warm person who will help ease the client's trepidation about seeing the therapist. The receptionist clearly contributes to the clinic's success and quality of services.

GREETING CLIENTS

Greet each client with enthusiasm and warmth. While in the waiting room, be sure that the client is offered amenities (e.g., water, soft drinks, magazines, or anything else—within reason—that they might need). Although they typically decline such offers, the beginnings of a bond, through your courtesy, are formed. They are likely not used to being treated with such care in a place of business. Any potential presuppositions or reservations they have about coming to therapy will likely be decreased. Make everyone feel welcome. If the receptionist is introverted, or untrained in greeting clients, role-play various situations. These skills can be learned.

Be sure to always maintain the confidentiality of clients' names. When a client enters the waiting area and other clients are also in the room, do not say their entire name. Typically, a first name is adequate. Do not have a sign-in sheet where the names of clients are visible to others signing in. Do your very best to be sure there is always someone available to greet and help clients, especially those there for a first time visit.

Greeting clients with a take-a-number mentality decreases the chance of repeat business. When clients arrive greet them by saying much more than "Do you have an appointment?" or "Have a seat." Likewise, do not be so overly friendly that it becomes intrusive to the client.

Do not immediately ask them for a co-payment. Although co-payments should be collected each visit, do not make it the first item on the agenda. The first item on the agenda is cordiality.

The client is likely tired of being unappreciated or taken for granted. The fact the he or she is coming to therapy may suggest

<hr />

Example of Not Respecting a Patient's Privacy

I recently brought my daughter to the hospital for a minor surgery. While in the waiting room a medical professional called a woman into an adjoining office. Her full name was called out. In addition, those sitting next to the extra room could easily hear the screening interview, during which she divulged information including her name, phone number, policy number, weight, height, and very personal physical concerns she was experiencing.

In mental health this would clearly constitute a breach of confidentiality and certainly embarrassment to the client.

<hr />

emptiness or need for acceptance. Show clients that you care and help them feel welcome. Make all efforts to set them at ease and ensure them their confidentiality will be preserved.

Train your office personnel to be courteous, professional, and people oriented. Provide ongoing staff training that includes role-playing various situations dealing with an array of client behaviors on the phone and in the waiting room. Additionally, include training in topics such as boundary issues, confidentiality, dealing with emergencies, and not providing advice to clients. Do not spare expenses in video training, seminars, or workshops designed to enhance customer service and professionalism. This relatively small investment yields a large reward.

Even though office personnel do not conduct therapy, do not assume that any relation building is solely practiced by the therapists. Hiring office personnel simply based on their administrative skills can be a costly error. Administrative skills will help certain aspects of the business run more smoothly, but personnel with crude people skills will likely lead to a loss of clientele. Do not assume that office personnel will not interact with clients.

Conversely, be sure that office personnel are sufficiently trained in boundary issues. Simply because someone works in a mental health clinic does not mean that he or she can offer advice or provide any type of therapy. Becoming overly familiar with clients can lead to ethical problems—not only for therapists, but also for office personnel. This could lead to staff socializing with clients, relationships, and attempts to look into client files—a definite ethical issue to the clinic. Without a staff policy and procedure handbook boundaries are murky.

Office workers who are efficient, but show poor people skills, might do more harm than good if they come in contact with clients. Some clients stop coming due to the behavior of nontherapists (e.g., receptionist, scheduler, billers, phone answering services). It is easier to lose a client than to keep a client.

CUSTOMER SERVICE TO REFERRAL SOURCES

Without a source of referrals it is impossible to sustain a clinic. Clients do not form a line for services once a practice opens its doors. Wise clinicians stay in regular contact with each of their referral sources. Outside agencies and professionals are very particular about where they send referrals. To them, making a referral is a reflection or extension of their work. They must have confidence that you will provide appropriate and helpful services. Even one client complaint could end a stream of referrals. Several other clinicians will line up happily to see these clients. Obtaining referrals is very competitive, requiring a set of skills similar to a public relations expert.

When you receive a referral always thank the referral source verbally, and/or in writing. An e-mail is too impersonal. A simple thank-you note, in your handwriting, goes a long way. Consider taking the referral source out to lunch to show your gratitude and to discuss other ways your agencies can be mutually helpful. However, never even hint at bribelike behaviors or become overindulgent to this person by providing incentives for referrals.

When you are in contact with a referred client, make an immediate and timely appointment. If at all possible, do not place this new client on a waiting list. Clearly communicate to the client what reports, if any, typically go to the referral source and how the information will be used. Always speak positively about the referral source to the client.

If you receive a referral for a specific purpose, do not provide additional services beyond the reason for the referral without a request from or a discussion with the referral source. This additional

Example of Customer Service to a Referral Source

Early in my career I specialized in providing group therapy to people with a dual-diagnosis of mild developmental delays and mental health or behavioral concerns. A number of therapists in the area also provided such services, but only a few of them communicated the results of the group therapy to the clients' treatment teams. Group home professionals stated that they were interested in what took place in the sessions in order to follow up on the group topics and individual needs.

A group syllabus was devised listing specific group topics a few months in advance. The group home staff and other providers were then aware of the focus of the group treatment. In addition, during every group session an intern or cotherapist would write a general outline of what took place in the group meeting (without other group members' names mentioned), plus another section of individual contributions where progress notes for the individual were noted. The individual's and the group's progress notes were then copied (with permission), with the original going into each group member's file, and copies sent to other providers of care. This sharing of information was extremely helpful in coordinating services. It also allowed for treatment teams to provide suggestions for future group topics.

The combination of an encompassing group outline and coordinated services helped the program grow to 12 groups of eight individuals within the first year of opening the practice. Fliers were sent to group homes and social workers who worked in the Developmental Disabilities Unit (Mental Retardation) of the county. The advertising included outlines of various upcoming groups focusing on issues such as depression, sexual issues, acting out, assertiveness, and other topics of interest. The response was strong because we provided very specific information concerning the group content and in the progress reports. (*Note:* If the client refused to allow reports to be shared with the treatment team, none were sent.)

The coordination of services involved some extra work; however, the increase in business was far beyond expectations. Many of the group clients also received individual services, and a regular stream of clients were referred to the clinic for other reasons, such as their required periodic evaluations for adaptive and intellectual functioning.

service might be in competition with the referral source, which could lead to the source viewing you as competing or stealing the client. When this takes place referrals end quickly, and your reputation among professionals could be damaged.

When you receive a referral, clearly discuss the specific reason for the referral. Find out what services the referral source is providing and specifically what they do and do not desire from you. For example if the referral is for testing only, do not offer the client counseling services if the source of the referral is a therapist. If the client receives individual therapy from another therapist who refers them to you for group therapy, do not provide individual therapy to the client unless the referral source requests it. It is much more difficult to regain lost trust than it is to initially build it.

THE IMPORTANCE OF YOUR PHYSICAL OFFICE REGARDING CUSTOMER SERVICE

The following information is in this chapter because the office location and décor are part of the overall customer service experienced by clients. However, this information also addresses some business aspects of your location.

Setting Up an Office

The location of your office will have an effect on the clientele who receive services at your clinic. Unfortunately, location has a price. Prime locations may be prestigious, but the rent may be prohibitive. Clients do not choose a therapist solely on location, but they may decide to use a clinic based on its location. Obviously, they will prefer a location that is convenient, but typically do not require a luxury suite.

Usually, for mental health clients, location is more about convenience than prestige. Factors to consider include clients' safety, clinic accessibility, cost of parking, traffic, distance, and traveling time. A suburban office may be more convenient for the therapist, but not necessarily for some clients.

When deciding on a location, set your priorities by considering three main factors: budget, client factors, and therapist factors. As mental health professionals we try to place our clients' needs first, but the reality is that we must live within a budget. Too many new practices go out of business rather quickly, and are then left owing the balance of a lease for several months. In many cases your budget narrows down the potential selections for your location.

Next, your clientele focus will help you select a location. Neighborhoods in both large and small cities usually differ by socioeconomic status, age, cultural groups, race, and several other demographic factors. Your areas of specialty will likely correspond with some neighborhoods or areas of the city more than others. If you work in a small town it might make little difference where you are located.

If, for example, you specialize in working with children, your best location might not be in an area where most people are at retirement age. Or, if you decide to only accept cash as payment, you will likely have difficulties in a low-income or poor neighborhood. Your certainly do not have to live near your clients, but make all efforts to work near them.

Leases

Once you have found a location where you would like to practice, search for office spaces that are for rent or for lease. Depending on the economy at the time, this task may be painless or bothersome. If there are a number of places competing for your business you will be able to negotiate a deal that works well for you. Some therapists prefer to look personally, while others use an agent.

When you look at office space keep in mind exactly what you need. Unless you are doing a fair amount of group work, do not pay for large offices. In a typical therapy situation, not much more is needed in a therapist's office than a desk, file cabinet, and a few chairs. A space of 8×8 or 8×10 feet is plenty of room for each therapist. In addition, you will need a waiting room and a lockable storage closet. If you plan on starting out as a sole practitioner two rooms and a closet are plenty of space. Therefore, when you look for

---

Example of Negotiating a Lease

My first independent practice was in an office building in Blaine, Minnesota. I had very little money, but plenty of motivation. I looked at about four places that were for lease. Three of them had been on the market for a brief period of time, while another one had been vacant for several months. The owners or managers of the three offices that were new on the market were not yet ready to negotiate. However, due to its apparent stagnancy, I decided that the office that had been available for a while would be a great opportunity for serious negotiations.

I told the owner that his office was perfect for me, but it needed some renovations to suit my needs. Since it doesn't hurt to ask, I proposed that I would do all of the renovations (i.e., painting and a few minor changes) if I could make no security deposit, plus have the first three months free of charge in a 1-year lease. In addition, I negotiated for a rent about 20 percent lower than the asking price. To my surprise, the owner, an attorney, agreed. I strongly suggest that you attempt to deal with the owner of the building, not an agent. In many instances, if they like you, and believe that you are stable, you will get a better deal (if you ask for it).

In my other location, I initially negotiated a graduated lease in which I agreed to eventually pay the quoted price, but not until the third year. The first 2 years I received a discount of 20 percent, then 10 percent, respectively.

Hint: A landlord will like you much more if you dwell on the benefits of his or her building. Do not pick on the flaws or he or she will likely become defensive. People will help out others who are trying to get started as long as they seem credible. However, not every landlord will negotiate. In such cases, unless you must have that office, walk away with your business card in their hand.

---

a place to rent, let them know that you are looking for only about 150 to 200 square feet to start out. Be sure to have a clause in your lease that allows you to upgrade to a larger space at the same price or less per square foot if you outgrow your space.

If you plan to stay at a location for at least a few years you might consider signing, for example, a 3-year lease. This will keep the payment at the rate of the first year for 3 years. Since a 3-year lease may be risky, especially for a new practice, offer the owner a graduated means of getting out of the lease in the contract. For example, if for some reason you must exit a 3-year lease during the first year, you will owe a buyout of 6 months; during the second year, a payment of 4 months; and during the last year, 2 months. This method protects your level of payment during the lease and protects you from paying the entire 3 years (if it is not re-rented or sublet-ted) if you are not able to stay in the office the full lease term.

One other item must be mentioned, to financially protect you. I do not provide legal advice, but I have found that working as a cor-poration protects you personally from any potential business liabil-ities. Some landlords will allow you to sign a lease in the name of a corporation, while others will allow it if you also sign personally. Carefully weigh the personal consequences of defaulting on a lease before you sign. When starting out, it is always more cautious to sign a short-term lease.

An office lease can either be a means of protecting the price you pay for rent, or it may lead to many financial problems. Owners of new practices must be careful when signing leases. A lease protects you from rent increases and eviction without good reason during the lease period. Leases are typically more negotiable when the of-fice space has been on the market for a while and when you are deal-ing directly with the owner, who is not being paid a commission like a broker.

If funds are short in the beginning, ask the landlord for a grad-uated lease, in which the monthly payment starts out small and gradually reaches the agreed-upon amount. Protect yourself by in-cluding clauses in the lease that leave you with the least amount of financial responsibility if you do need to vacate early.

Without a lease the landlord can ask you to vacate in 30 days at any time. Basically, a no-lease agreement is a month-to-month lease in which either party can end the transaction after any given month. The landlord can, at will, increase your lease amount with a 30-day notice.

Be careful before signing a long-term lease, because many mental health practices go out of business within a year due to lack of business acumen. For example, if you sign a three-year lease for $800 per month, and must leave the location after 1 year, you could owe the landlord almost $20,000 if no one sublets or negotiates a lease with the landlord that ends your lease agreement.

Furniture/Décor

A therapist's office does not have to be exorbitant. Simple furnishings are always in good taste. Although you will never please everyone, try to choose color schemes and furnishings that would not be considered distasteful or offensive. At the same time, reflect your personality and individuality.

Used office furniture stores typically have very high quality, well-designed furniture. It is typically much more sturdy and professional looking than home furniture or inexpensive new furniture. Prices are also negotiable, and often less than one half to one fourth of the price when new.

Decorate the office in a manner suggesting warmth and cleanliness. The office environment is a representation of the therapist and the profession to the client. If furniture is shabby there could be an association with shabby therapy or a lack of caring. Stylish, well-coordinated furnishings represent order and careful planning and might suggest how the clinic feels about its clients. The choice of warm versus cool colors clearly sets different atmospheres.

I used to decorate with neutral colors such as white or beige in my offices. No one ever commented about the colors. However, when homier colors replaced the neutrals, several clients remarked that they felt more relaxed and comfortable.

Recently, I leased one of my offices to another professional, who wanted to use the space on the days I was in a different location. She subsequently put up a number of nature pictures in the waiting room, including images of wolves chasing deer. Immediately, a few clients questioned why a therapist's waiting room would have pictures depicting violence. It was difficult because she was quite fond of them, but I asked her to please remove the pictures. Fortunately, she complied and the original scenic pictures were replaced.

The surroundings and décor of an office clearly set a tone of either warmth or coldness. Furnishings such as pictures and posters should be in good, or at least neutral, taste to most people. Consider the wide range of your clients' political, religious, and cultural beliefs and boundaries when choosing office décor. What is neutral to one person could be offensive to another.

One therapist tried hanging a wide variety of posters on the wall that expressed various words of wisdom. One poster quoted a religious source. A client, on his first visit to the clinic, walked out because he was offended, believing that the clinic was going to push their religious beliefs on him. Not everyone will be pleased all of the time, but careful consideration should be taken to not offend people due to artwork, posters, or other means of expression.

An inviting, peaceful, and clean environment says much about the clinic, and it helps prepare the client for counseling. Although you may express yourself artistically however you desire, try to make all attempts to avoid offending clients with your décor. Décor that suggests both professionalism and serenity seem to be the best match. Professionalism can be depicted with items including mental health posters with positive themes, lists of professional services, ethics statements, or copies of your therapists' licenses. Themes of serenity are easily displayed through color, artwork, and lighting.

Security / Safety / Accessibility

Do not set up an office in an unsafe area. This does not mean that there should be no mental health treatment clinics in certain areas of a city. It means that if your practice is in a high crime area, take all precautions to protect your clients' safety. For example, a parking lot with little or no lighting can lead to an unsafe situation. If you live in a cold climate be sure sidewalks are shoveled when it snows.

Be sure your building is safe. Stairways should have railings. Adequate protection such as fire extinguishers, smoke alarms, and security cameras are very helpful. Do not lease or purchase an office that is not handicap accessible.

SUMMARY

Answer the telephone immediately whenever possible. Whether the phone is being answered by a therapist, answering service, or a receptionist, be sure the person answering is able to answer a variety of questions about the therapists and the clinic, plus schedule appointments. Keep track of commonly asked questions and have answers prepared.

Do not rely on voice mail or answering machines for most phone calls, especially during regular business hours. If you do, you will certainly lose business. Unless the phone call is a previous client or a very strong referral, making an appointment with you is no different to the client than the next therapist's name on the list. Most of these missed referrals will be lost to other clinics. We are living in an "I want it now" society. Clients do not want to wait for a call back to arrange an appointment. It is often too stressful.

Answering services may not be as good as an on-site employee, but some services can leave a positive impression about the clinic. Although it is usually not possible, try to work out an arrangement that allows the answering service to schedule appointments, or at least make a tentative appointment until the therapist confirms it. Without such an arrangement many referrals will be lost when clients phone another clinic.

Treat each referral source as if your well-being depended on it, because it does. When someone makes a referral to you they are doing you a favor and you are helping their client. Treat them likewise. Keep in constant communication. Regularly ask them if there is anything you can do differently to better suit their needs. Never say or do anything that would harm the relationship, unless there are ethical reasons it should be ended. Find out what other clinics are doing when they receive a referral, and then do more. You have been chosen for referrals for a reason. Find out why referrals are sent to you and continue the practice.

Let referral sources know that you are available for questions. When referral sources view you as a valuable resource their referrals will continue. When they contact you, happily speak with them about their questions. Be available to speak to groups at their place of business. Referrals will increase if you maintain this type of service.

If you take referrals for granted, or begin to expect them, they will cease. Lack of contact with your referral sources suggests they mean little to you. Referral sources do not come out of the blue; you must actively seek them. Without this extra effort, growth will be slow or nil.

Referral sources place much trust in you. They are typically putting their clients in your hands; thus, the quality of your services reflects on them. They expect that their clients will receive exceptional service from you; otherwise, they would not have made the referral. Referrals are the backbone of a clinic and must be treated accordingly. Show them your heartfelt appreciation.

The location of your office affects who will be your clientele. Make all efforts to locate your office in the vicinity of your preferred clientele. Choose a location convenient for public transportation, parking, handicap accessibility, and other services in the area. Try to locate your office near stores or similar places for people waiting for your clients. Many people do not want to sit in the waiting room while you are seeing clients. An office near a county human services building may attract referrals from county case managers. An office near an attorney's office is convenient for referrals involving legal matters.

When an office has cheap rent there is a reason. Oftentimes the office's location is a contributing factor. A poor location will cause a decrease in business. For example, clientele who do not drive or have access to a ride may not want to take a bus if the nearest bus stop is over a few blocks away. Or, if parking is a problem, so that clients must either pay a high price or walk too far from their car due to a lack of parking spaces, they are likely to discontinue using your clinic due to the inconvenience.

TEST YOUR KNOWLEDGE

1. If a clinic is very busy and no appointments are available for at least a few weeks, what is usually the best course of action, according to this book?

    (a) Place the person on a waiting list.

    (b) Refer the client to another provider.

    (c) Immediately hire a new therapist.

    (d) Place the person in a group.

2. Answering machines are an excellent means of taking messages, but they

   (a) are very helpful in a clinic.

   (b) are better than an answering service.

   (c) should be used in a clinic because therapists shouldn't answer the phone.

   (d) may lead to lost business in a clinic.

3. An answering service is most effective when it

   (a) simply takes basic information and relays it to the clinic.

   (b) provides clinical advice to clients in emergency situations.

   (c) is able to provide a level of information similar to a receptionist.

   (d) lets clients know that someone will get back to them soon.

4. Matching clients to therapists

   (a) should only be handled by experienced professionals.

   (b) should be solely at the client's discretion.

   (c) can be handled by an adequately trained receptionist.

   (d) requires hours of matching client and therapist variables.

5. The location of your office

   (a) is not important because clients will travel if you are an excellent therapist.

   (b) is very important when clients look for services.

   (c) should be in a busy part of the city.

   (d) should be near your home.

Answers: 1. b; 2. d; 3. c; 4. c; 5. b

3

Obtaining Third-Party Contracts and Working with Managed Care

In my experience, several changes have taken place in a number of managed care companies. About 10 to 15 years ago, many therapists became quite irritated with managed care companies because it was difficult to get on those companies' panels. And, if they became a provider, a low number of services were allowed for their clients. It was not uncommon to be required to request authorization for additional sessions for clients every few appointments. Each time services were requested, the therapist would have to contact a case manager to discuss the case. Oftentimes the therapist would be on hold for lengthy periods of time. It simply wasn't worth it.

As time has gone on and reforms have taken place, managed care, in general, is more user friendly to therapists. Most managed care companies have significantly extended the number of sessions allowed before an authorization is required and have made the authorization process more streamlined. Positive changes have taken place, but many therapists still avoid managed care.

BECOMING A PROVIDER

Sooner of later most therapists are faced with the decision of whether to become a provider for various insurance companies. Depending on the type of clinic, becoming an insurance provider may or may not be necessary. If a clinic's source of revenue, for example, is through state or county contracts, being an insurance provider might not be necessary. Some clinics receive funds through donations or nonprofit funding. However, it is not possible that all clinics can be funded by government or private sources. The primary source of clients for most private practices is individuals with insurance, which is typically provided through a managed care contract. Because of this fact, very few mental health clinics survive without third-party contracts.

A negative aspect of working with managed care is providers accepting a lower fee for services. But you will save in advertising expenses because they provide you with referrals. There has been a fair amount of negative press about managed care. Profit margins and reimbursements have often led to public outcry. However, there have been positive changes, and much good has come out of managed care. This text is not intended to side with or against managed care, but, rather, it will discuss how to be accepted by, excel in, and remain on managed care panels for those who wish to become providers.

It is difficult to make blanket statements about managed care insurance because the quality of services available to recipients of these policies varies. The reader is advised to discuss various insurance providers with local professionals who are on the panels of managed care companies. Thus, the following information is generic, but should hold true in most instances and in most geographical areas.

In some regions, becoming an insurance provider is very competitive. Some private practices have gone out of business because clients had to go somewhere else that accepted their insurance. Unfortunately, many therapists have applied to become a provider but have been turned down because "the network is full." I have heard many therapists complain that they cannot obtain managed care contracts. The following sections will provide steps to increase one's chances of becoming a provider.

STEPS TO OBTAIN MANAGED CARE CONTRACTS

Step 1: Research the Company

Some managed care providers are more therapist-friendly than others. The level of payment, rejection rates, services covered, documentation required, number of potential clients, and level of difficulty receiving an authorization for payment can vary significantly. Some companies pay well and are therapist-friendly. They make the process of setting up an appointment uncomplicated, and their billing and payment processes are streamlined and straightforward. They have case managers readily available to answer questions and approve procedures. Their policies and procedures leave few gray areas.

Other managed care companies make it very difficult for clients to receive services. Their payment rate can be so low that a therapist would have to see a bulk number of clients to be financially worthwhile. Usually, the telephone time spent on hold discourages the therapist from communicating, resulting in denial of services. Some companies do not pay for report writing time or time spent explaining findings to the client.

Before considering becoming a provider, carefully research the benefits and drawbacks of the third-party payer. Typically, the best feedback you can receive is from other therapists. There is an array of questions that would be helpful to ask your peers prior to becoming a provider for a particular company. If you do not know a therapist who is a provider for an insurance company, ask the company for a list of providers. Then contact a provider and let them know your concerns over lunch. Ask questions such as the following:

1. Overall, what is your opinion of the company?

2. How is their customer service?

3. How many sessions do they initially approve?

4. What paperwork do they require to obtain additional services?

5. What is their hourly payment rate?

6. Do they pay for report writing time?

7. How often do they refer clients to you?

8. Can you bill them online?

9. Are their policies and procedures straightforward?

10. Do they cover relationship counseling?

11. What percentage of claims do they reject?

12. What are their typical reasons for rejecting claims?

13. What is the typical waiting time for payment?

14. Can a certain number of sessions take place before an authorization is needed?

15. Do they charge an administrative fee to become a provider?

Step 2: The Application Process

Some insurance providers have their own applications, while others use a universal application form. In competitive markets where it is difficult to obtain managed care contracts, your application must stand out above the rest. This does not necessarily mean that the application itself must be more visibly noticeable (e.g., bright, colored paper), but rather the content and specificity of services are most important when a third-party payer reviews applications to become a provider.

All applications look the same, therefore it is important to provide information that others typically do not include. For example, sending an addendum that contains a sample client file including the intake, treatment plan, progress notes, billing, and discharge summary provide an excellent opportunity to demonstrate the quality of both your therapy and documentation. Of course, do not include any information that would identify the client.

Managed care companies are also interested in good customer service. Emphasize on your application aspects such as a wide range of hours to see clients, handicapped accessibility, convenience of your location, and how quickly you can see new clients. Policies such as same-day appointments for emergencies and a waiting list of no longer than 1 week for a regular appointment speaks wonders.

Third-party payers routinely require that providers have professional liability insurance. The usual requirement is called a $1 million/$3 million policy. Do not wait to purchase liability insurance until you have received managed care contracts. You likely will not receive contracts without it, and even without such contracts, liability insurance is a must. Most professional organizations have contracts for special rates available for members.

Managed care companies are very particular about the therapist's record of ethics violations, professional complaints, license suspensions, and other profession concerns that may suggest a higher potential for liability. The applications contain some very specific and personal questions. If you have had some ethical concerns, professional complaints, or liability issues, be sure to clearly disclose the information and discuss how you resolved the issues. Most applications to become a provider include the following types of information:

Copy of current license	College degrees
Practice location(s) and hours	Internship and postgraduate training
Clinical specialty areas	Employment history
Population of ages served	Vita
Proof in liability insurance	Professional affiliations
Requests for transcripts	Professional references
Billing information	Hospital affiliations
Disclosure of ethical complaint issues	Immunity information

In competitive markets, do not be discouraged by an initial rejection. I practice in a very competitive market for managed care contracts. Some contracts were obtained after the first application, while others took three or four tries. If you are initially rejected for a contract, try to find out the reason for the rejection. A typical cover rejection letter will usually state that the panel is full and they will keep your application on file. Do not simply wait to hear from them. If possible, discuss the application with a case manager or someone who is involved in approving contracts. Most therapists simply give up, but those who persist have a much greater chance of being accepted in a subsequent application. In the meantime, find out what provisions are made for a *nonpreferred provider.* A nonpreferred provider may bill an insurance company, but typically the client's copayment is higher.

In mental health treatment, there is an abundance of either generalists or those who provide only a very narrow range of services. A generalist likely has a lesser chance of obtaining a contract because of the abundance of generalists. Clients do not ask for a therapist who is a generalist. The one-size-fits-all mentality does not work well in mental health treatment. Emphasize specific areas of your experience and training that are typically not found in other clinics. Do not simply note this on their checklist, but also include it in your cover letter. Examples of competencies commonly found in managed care applications are included in the following.

Example List of Competencies in Managed Care Applications

List of competencies that will be used to inform patients of the services you provide. Check the services in which you are trained and provide.

__ Abuse: Sexual/Physical/Emotional	__ Grief counseling
__ ADHD evaluations	__ Group therapy
__ ADHD treatment	__ Home-based counseling services
__ Adjustment Disorders	__ Hypnosis
__ Affective Disorders	__ Marriage and family counseling
__ Anxiety Disorders	__ Mental Retardation
__ Asperger	__ Neuropsychological evaluations
__ Autism	__ OCD
__ Biofeedback	__ Personality Disorders
__ Bipolar	__ Panic Disorder/Agoraphobia
__ CD evaluations	__ Psychotic Disorders
__ CD treatment	__ Medical management
__ Couples	__ Pain Disorder
__ Crisis counseling	__ Psychological evaluations
__ Dialectical Behavioral Training	__ PTSD
__ Dual Dx MICD	__ Religious/spiritual counseling
__ Dissociate Disorders	__ Sexual Disorders
__ Eating Disorders	__ Severe, chronic mental illness
__ Family therapy	__ Other _____
__ Gay/lesbian	__ Other _____

There are times of the year when mental health clinics tend to be busiest and clients must wait longer to obtain an appointment. Thus, there is a higher likelihood of obtaining a contract during these busy times. Suggested times of applying are January through March and September through early November. However, some companies accept providers only at specific times when there are scheduled committee meetings.

An application usually inquires about the therapist's therapeutic stance. This text is not intended to suggest a particular mode of therapy; however, short-term therapy models tend to be more preferred due to the cost savings to the payer. If you list that you specialize in an experimental model or only provide long-term therapy, there is a lesser chance of being placed on a preferred provider list.

This is not to say that all clients will receive short-term therapy. The point is to inform the provider that you are proficient in both short-term and long-term therapy. Certain problem areas may take a considerable amount of time to work through. But, if your application suggests that you see most clients for long periods of time, rejection is more likely. Most therapeutic schools of thought have both short-term and long-term applications. Become familiar with the average number of sessions and most effective treatments for various diagnoses and problem areas. Briefly relay your knowledge of such information in your cover letter.

Before you apply for any managed care panels, first become a provider for both Medicare (federal) and Medicaid (state). Most applications for managed care ask for your provider number for each of these funding sources. If you do not have them, it might suggest that you have little experience. Becoming a provider for Medicare and Medicaid is not competitive, so you should be able to become a provider with little or no difficulty.

When you apply to become a provider for any third party, be patient. You will not receive an approval in a few weeks. Many times the process can take a few months. There is very little you can do to speed up the process. The procedure is lengthy because they must check your references, insurance, and educational transcripts, and evaluate the need for your specific services, plus wait until one or more committees meet for the final decision. Even once you are approved, a final committee signature is needed after you have signed the contract. This may take an additional month. It is not unusual to wait 3 to 4 months until you may see their clients.

Be sure that the application is completely filled out. It is possible that you could fill out an application and receive a reply several weeks later informing you that the application is not complete. It will not go any further until you act. This causes a significant time delay. They do not act upon incomplete applications. In addition, be sure that your references respond to their inquiries, and double check that transcripts and insurance verifications have been received. It is a good idea to phone the managed care company to verify that all application materials have been received.

REMAINING A PROVIDER

Becoming a provider and remaining a provider depend primarily on customer service, therapeutic skills, ethics, and documentation. Managed care contracts are typically renewed on a yearly basis. The renewal application is similar to the initial application, but reviewed with less scrutiny, unless there has been a history of complaints, excessive billing practices, ethical issues, or other factors suggesting decreased competency. Items such as a licensure renewal certificate, proof of liability insurance, and a renewed list of competencies are typically required.

SUMMARY

Be sure to fill out all of the information requested in an application. If possible, when applying to be an insurance provider, type the application. Provide a full list of services and emphasize the convenience and helpfulness of your practice. Include addendums to the application that allow you to stand out in a professional manner. Do not be discouraged if your application is rejected the first time. Persistence pays off. Get the point across that you can handle general counseling concerns and that you are competent in one or more specialty areas (e.g., DBT, Christian counseling, Mental Retardation, domestic abuse, Pain Disorders, ADHD, group therapy, neuropsychological evaluations).

Do not overstate your qualifications. Unless you have definite training and supervision, do not claim to be competent in those areas. Do not hide any concerns such as malpractice suits or ethical complaints because this is often public information.

An application that appears to be hastily written will likely be hastily reviewed. If you do not carefully and specifically answer each question, you leave room for doubt.

Managed care contracts can generate a great deal of business in a clinic. In the past, some clinics would spend up to several hundred dollars per month for *Yellow Page* ads, but most insurance clients choose from their provider manual rather than *The Yellow Pages* because they see only the professionals listed, rather than choosing the clinic with the largest ad.

Being on a provider panel is typically an effortless way to obtain referrals. They will contact you, not because they have heard about your services, but because you are the preferred provider. As you develop rapport with the case managers at the managed care company, you will likely see even more referrals sent your way.

Working with managed care typically involves increased paperwork and a requirement to follow specific procedures, which vary from company to company. The medical model of documentation is the norm. It is extremely important to learn documentation procedures (see Chapter 11). The number of sessions you provide is not unlimited, and you must empirically demonstrate the medical necessity to provide additional services. If you see a very high number of clients, you increase your chances for an audit. The hourly fee is typically about 80 percent of the usual and customary fees charged in your area.

Therapists who see a wide variety of clients for many diagnoses and problem areas have the potential to see many clients. They rarely refer clients to others because of the universality of their approach. Indeed if they are able to help a wide range of clients, they are an asset to any clinic. Typically, they work best in an outpatient practice where most of their clients are experiencing mild to moderate mental health symptoms due to a reaction to a current stressor. Being a generalist can be very helpful, but it is equally helpful to learn at least one specialty. A specialist may do quite well in a managed care setting due to case managers providing them with referrals. However, some specialty areas receive an abundance of referrals, while others are rarely needed or trendy.

Although generalists may do well helping people with non-threatening mental health issues, they might not be prepared to deal with clients with chronic and persistent mental health dysfunction. Specific clinical understanding and therapeutic techniques are needed and will help when applying for third-party contracts. Unless a specialist provides a service that is in fairly high demand, the therapist must have other competencies to fill in the time slots when not practicing the specialty. For example, if a therapist only sees male, teenaged clients with bulimia and practices in a small town, it will be very difficult to work a full-time schedule.

It is fine to practice as either a generalist or a specialist, but the business of mental health is market driven. It is wise for therapists to investigate what the mental health treatment needs of their community are and obtain and receive appropriate training and education in areas related to their interests and capabilities. Learning a specialty in which there are few potential clients certainly may help a few clients but may not take care of the therapist's financial needs. Obtaining training as both a generalist and in a specialty area would likely best prepare a clinician for a variety of career possibilities.

TEST YOUR KNOWLEDGE

1. What is the greatest advantage of becoming a provider for a managed care company?

    (a) You collect a higher fee per client.

    (b) You have an unlimited number of sessions.

    (c) You receive referrals from them.

    (d) You receive kickbacks for limiting the number of sessions.

2. When applying for a managed care contract it is suggested that you emphasize

   (a) both generalist and specialist competencies.

   (b) your attributes as a generalist.

   (c) your attributes as a specialist.

   (d) your low cost for services.

3. If you apply for a managed care contract and are turned down because "the network is full,"

   (a) accept the decision and go on.

   (b) phone them and ask for an appointment.

   (c) try again.

   (d) contact the insurance commissioner in your state.

4. Competency in clinical proficiency is based on

   (a) education.

   (b) supervision.

   (c) experience.

   (d) all of these.

Answers: 1. c; 2. a; 3. c; 4. d

4

Other Means of Obtaining Referrals

Mental health clinics do not stand on their own; they must have referral sources. There is clearly no gold bricked road leading to your place of business. A thriving clinic depends on referral sources. This writer spends at least an hour per week *working referrals*. That is, at least one hour per week is devoted to finding new business or contacting existing referral sources. It is far too time consuming to knock on the door of every potential referral source. But, if they have never heard of you, exposure is needed.

As in any other business, there are vendors and consumers. The consumer must decide which vendor to use from a list of several who are in competition with each other. When people go shopping they typically have some idea of what product they are looking for, and what they are willing to pay. If they go to a store and the product is not available, of low quality, or the store does not accept their method of payment, they will go elsewhere. Likewise, if a clinic does not offer the appropriate services to fit clients' needs, or does not accept their insurance, they will go elsewhere. A clinic director/manager must keep track of what services the public desires, plus have the receptionist monitor the number of referrals to the clinic that are turned down or referred to others due to the service not being available. If a clinic loses a fair amount of business due to not accepting certain insurances, it is a good idea to consider becoming a provider, when appropriate.

OBTAINING REFERRALS

Referrals rarely come from the sign outside of your building. Each referral takes a fair amount of work, and may come from a variety of sources. A new clinic does not have the benefit of receiving referrals from previous clients. As the clinic grows, less effort is needed in actively advertising for referrals, due to referrals stemming from previous clients. The following examples constitute a number of methods for expanding a mental health business.

MAILERS / BROCHURES

One of the greatest sources of obtaining referrals is through mailers to other professionals who have contact with people who need mental health services. A professional-quality brochure (glossy, colored pictures, well-written, concise) creates a great first impression. A black-and-white flier fresh off the copy machine will usually do more harm than good. Both high and low quality are easy to recognize. A professional-quality brochure will be associated with a high-quality clinic. Sending out regular mailers can be fairly expensive, but the rate of return can be abundant.

Purchasing glossy, colored brochures from a printing company is quite expensive. One brochure may cost in the vicinity of 30¢ or more in bulk. Thus, a mailer to 1,000 addresses will cost over $700 when calculating the brochure, postage, and other related costs. However, it does not have to be that expensive for the same quality work. Consider the following:

1. Purchase a professional-quality color laser printer. This is the biggest initial expense, but it will last for a number of years. Typically, an excellent printer that retails for close to $5,000 can be purchased on the Internet for not much over $3,000. This is an excellent investment if you mean business and want to become aggressive in advertising.

2. Learn a desktop publishing program. Be sure that the one you purchase is compatible with the printer. This is not as much of an issue as it has been in the past. Typically, even the least expensive desktop publishing programs are capable of producing an excellent-looking brochure. With today's level of user friendliness and the tutorials available, it does not take much time to learn to use such programs. Many community colleges offer one- or two-day seminars to teach desktop publishing.

3. Contact several area clinics and ask them to send you a brochure. They will give you as many ideas on what to do, as what not to do. They will also provide you with information as to what services they offer (and do not offer).

4. Brochure writing is a talent in itself. It is very tempting to provide far too much information. However, readers like graphics and text that is informative but not exhausting. A bold heading with five or six bulleted points is far more likely to be read than a paragraph. Too much text ends up in the basket. Likewise, too many graphics may seem juvenile or nonprofessional. For example: Which of the following is easier for you to read: A or B?

Example A: Poor Example of Clinic Information in a Brochure

The XYZ clinic specializes in individual therapy for adults and children. We have 12 therapists with degrees in social work, psychology, professional counseling, and marriage and family therapy. Our therapists have experience ranging from 2 to 20 years in the field. We work with clients suffering from depression, anxiety, eating disorders, learning problems, ADHD, OCD, conduct problems, oppositional behaviors, adjustment issues, coping problems, pain disorders, and relationship issues. Our fees are based on your ability to pay, plus we accept most insurances. Our hours of operation are Monday through Thursday, 9 AM to 9 PM, and Friday through Saturday, 9 AM to 3 PM. Emergency services are available. We provide a variety of therapies, including cognitive-behavioral, psychoanalytic, client-centered, and solutions-focused treatment. Both short-term and long-term therapy are available. We have female and male therapists on staff. We are able to refer to a psychiatrist. We have someone on call 24 hours per day. Each therapist is fully licensed and insured. Our clinic is accredited by Joint Commission of Accredited Health Organizations. Services are available within 1 week. You will find us to be warm, compassionate, and understanding. We are here because we care.

Example B: Good Example of Clinic Information in a Brochure

(Picture of a relaxed client with a therapist in comfortable surroundings)

At XYZ clinic you have a choice of . . .

Several caring therapists from a wide variety of backgrounds and expertise.

Day, evening, or Saturday hours.

Professional treatment that best fits your needs.

Insurance plans and sliding scale fees available.

Together. . . . Hand-in-hand. . . . In your time of need.

Discussion of Examples A and B

Example A provides much more information than Example B, but it is lengthy and boring in its 198 words. It talks about the clinic, not the individual who needs services. It is likely that the passage will not be read in its entirety. Much of the information it contains is expected in a mental health clinic. There is no emotion in the writing, just statements about services. If the prospective reader is someone with current emotional problems, it does little to provide a sense of hope and caring at the clinic.

Example B contains only 44 words (24 percent of Example A), but combined with the graphic, sense of caring, emotionality, and focus on the client, it is a much better advertisement. The text is easy to read and the spacing allows time to focus. It speaks volumes more than Example A. Rather than talking about what the clinic does, it highlights the client's needs (e.g., you, your). Much of the other information contained in Example A is not that important to the client, or is simply expected at a good mental health clinic.

A client suffering from emotional concerns is best reached emotionally. The graphic above the writing should portray a sense of caring, human-to-human togetherness, and calmness in a professional setting. Clients will envision themselves in that picture. You have reached them in more ways than simply reading a long paragraph. This is not manipulating people, but reaching them. *A picture is worth a thousand words.*

What to Include in a Clinic Brochure

The above example fits best in a clinic where the focus of treatment is on emotional or coping problems. The example would not work very well if your specialty is child behavior problems, neuropsychological evaluations, or any type of treatment that does not deal primarily with affective concerns.

Tailor your brochure to your intended clientele. It is not uncommon for a clinic to have several brochures, each with a different intended audience. For example, there would be separate brochures describing programs for children, adolescents, adults, groups, evaluations, and so forth. Once you learn desktop publishing, the only additional cost is the time to be creative in writing a brochure. Actually, it can be quite fun, and an escape from your usual routine.

Because brochures are an exercise in creativity, stipulating a specific format in this text would be stifling. However, a few elements are suggested. Most brochures are tri folded. The reader immediately sees the front and back cover (with focus on the front) before it is opened. Carefully choose the wording and graphics for the front cover. This first impression will determine if the brochure is read or discarded. Make sure that it matches the needs and expectations of the intended readership.

The following suggestions are made for the various readerships of your brochures.

Readership	Suggestions
Professionals	Do not write an emotionally laden brochure. It is intended to enumerate the services, professionalism, convenience, and customer services of your clinic. However, do not make it so sterile that even the professional reading it will become bored. Highlight your professional qualifications and describe how your services will benefit the other professional and the client. Do not write it as

if you are God's gift to the profession, but emphasize service and professionalism. Use several bullets, rather than lengthy paragraphs.

Parents/Caregivers	Emphasize specific behavioral issues that you treat in therapy of disruptive children. For example, do not simply say, we treat disruptive behaviors, children with Oppositional Defiance Disorder (ODD), Conduct Disorder, and ADHD—the reader may have never heard of these diagnoses. Parents and caregivers relate more to specific behavior problems and symptoms. For example, listings of the *symptoms* of diagnoses such as ODD, Conduct Disorder, and ADHD provide good descriptions. Do not list all of the symptoms, but enough to describe typical concerns for specific problem behaviors. Consider beginning the brochure with a question such as, "Does your child have difficulty in any of these areas?"

Defiant toward adults	Disruptive at school
Refuses to cooperate	Easily distracted
Cannot pay attention	Usually "on the go"
Lies, cheats, steals, bullies	Loses or does not do homework

Adults with emotional concerns	As in Example B the key is to reach the person in need emotionally. Get the message across that she or he is the focus. The graphics and pictures are important in relaying a sense of calmness

and hope without being too airy or over-indulgent. Statements such as, "We provide hope to the hopeless and love to the loveless," have no place in a professional brochure.

Psychological evaluations

Referrals for psychological evaluations typically come from other professionals, rather than the client. Typical sources for referrals include schools, social workers, courts, vocational rehabilitation staff, group homes, foster care, worker's compensation, disability funding sources, forensic sources, other mental health professionals, attorneys, employers, and social service agencies. The format of the brochure works well when it is written specifically for each group. A general brochure for psychological evaluations is too vague. Thus, separating brochures for each group and focusing on their specific needs is suggested. If you have desktop publishing capabilities and a professional color laser printer, revising one to another does not take much time. If each brochure is produced by outside sources, it could be cost prohibitive. Brochures with titles such as the following are helpful.

Psychological Evaluations for (any of these or others):

Developmental Delays	Mental Health
Employment screening	Behavioral Disorders
Learning Disabilities	ADHD
Neuropsychometric testing	Forensic evaluations
Disability evaluations	CD evaluations

What to Do with the Brochures

Brochures are somewhat effective in the office if clients distribute them, but since the clients are already at your office, the brochure they are reading is likely not the reason they made the appointment. Brochures are best utilized as mailers. The question is, "To whom do I mail the brochures?" There are numerous mailing lists available. Some are free and others must be paid for. Most mailing lists can be found on the Internet for free with a fair amount of searching.

Examples of where to find free mailing lists (which will vary from state to state).

Client Concern	Source of Mailing List
Mental Retardation	**1.** Ask the county for a list of social workers in the DD or MR unit. Then, send them brochures of your services. To save postage, bring all of them to the county building and ask the receptionist to distribute them in the social workers' mailboxes.
	2. Look on the Internet for group homes in the geographic areas you are interested in. Licensed facilities are often listed.
	3. Look on the Internet or in *The Yellow Pages* for social service agencies. Cross reference for the particular group you are interested in.
	4. Conduct an Internet search for "professional mailing lists" or "mental health mailing lists." Several companies will appear. Various companies specialize in lists that appeal to mental health clinics.
Mental health and mental behavior problems	**1.** Contact the county mental health unit. A list of social workers should be available. If they do not provide their

names bring in or send a packet of brochures to the unit, and request that they be distributed to the social workers focusing on mental health.

2. Physicians who might provide referrals for mental health are typically primary care and family physicians. Their names or respective clinics can be found through *The Yellow Pages,* an Internet search, licensing boards, or mailing list companies.

Group therapy

1. Mental health professional lists are obtainable from several sources, including state licensure boards and mailing list companies. It is much less expensive to obtain lists of clinics, rather than lists of individual therapists, because there are fewer clinics than therapists. That is, several therapists are likely to work in a single clinic, and one brochure can be distributed among all of them.

2. Group therapy brochures that include the agenda of the intended group have been successful when sent to county social workers.

Practice making several brochures, and ask colleagues for feedback. Your first effort will likely take several hours. But, the learning curve is very steep. Decide upon an overall format that stands out, but does not stick out.

Be consistent in your brochures. Keep certain elements such as fonts, graphics, and logos the same. Readers will associate them with your clinic. However, do not repeatedly send the same brochure. Make changes that preserve the consistency of previous brochures, but add new information. Otherwise, your brochures will become too commonplace and will be ignored.

Send out brochures on a regular basis, such as every few months, at least at first. This will keep the clinic fresh in the mind of the reader. Do not become discouraged if you do not hear from potential referral sources after several brochures have been sent. Just keep sending them. Many referrals come indirectly as the result of a brochure, so we do not always know where they originated. A brochure could change hands a few times before it is used.

A good return rate on any mailer is two to three percent. That is, if you send out 100 brochures and receive two responses, you are doing well. The other 98 recipients have some exposure to your services and they might remember something about you the next time they receive a brochure. Mere exposure and name recognition are an important aspect of advertising. For example, if a potential referral source has received several brochures from you over the years, perhaps one day someone might ask him or her, "Does anyone know where they have anger management groups?" Your name will likely come up if the referral source has been exposed to it enough. Each mailer you send adds to your exposure and his or her memory of the services you have to offer.

When someone responds to your brochure, be sure to ask if he or she would like a packet of brochures and business cards for distribution to other professionals at his or her place of business. Also, be sure that you follow through with every item mentioned in the brochure. It is better to understate than overstate your qualifications.

COUNTY CASEWORKERS

County social workers (or caseworkers) are typically the gatekeepers to mental health services for their clients. A larger county may have a group of several social workers working in several different units. Typical units may include children's mental health, adult mental health, developmental disabilities, child protection, foster care, financial workers, intake workers, and others. Developing relationships with county social workers can lead to consistent referrals.

As stated previously, you do not have to worry about the cost of postage if you bring in one brochure for every county social worker who works with clients in your specialty area. Simply ask the department secretary to please distribute them in their boxes. If it is not convenient to personally bring brochures, many counties will supply you with a list of the names of each social worker, and their respective unit. It is always a good idea to include a cover letter with each brochure. Create brochures that fit the needs of the clientele in each unit.

I have had excellent results with brochures. Even though brochures typically go to the same people, each time a mailer is sent out new referrals come in. Whenever my referrals begin to decrease, a new batch of revised brochures are sent out. Internet searches are regularly conducted to discover new referral sources. The exploration and the creativity involved provide a welcome outlet.

Another means of receiving referrals from social workers is to ask to speak briefly at their unit meeting. Prepare a presentation outlining your services. You do not have to emphasize how competent you are as a therapist; they expect that. Rather, emphasize availability, service, and communication. They highly appreciate periodic summary reports of the effects of therapy, along with recommendations and any efforts you make to coordinate treatment with other providers. That is, let them know that you want to be part of the client's treatment team, rather than providing unnecessary or duplicate services. Let them know that their input and feedback are important to successful therapy.

When you receive a referral from a county social worker or case-manager, do not simply take the referral and never contact the referral source again. Prior to seeing the client, clearly communicate with the referral source and the client what level of information will be shared throughout treatment. The better the quality of communication with referral sources, the greater chance of future referrals.

Some potential referral sources do not refer clients because they do not know the benefits of mental health services. In such cases, *create the need*. That is, educate them on the benefits of your services and how they will help both them and their clients. Provide examples of your work such as sample reports, treatment plans, progress reports, group outlines, or any other means of showing what can be expected from your services. However, do not make any promises that you cannot fulfill.

GROUP HOMES AND TREATMENT CENTERS

Group homes and treatment centers are similar in that clients live there either permanently or temporarily while receiving professional care. Clients receive these services for a variety of reasons, including chemical dependency, mental health issues, developmental delays, low adaptive functioning, effects of brain injuries, family issues, physical disabilities, effects of aging, and more. Web searches for items such as "CD treatment centers (your state)," "licensed foster care facilities (your state)," "residential treatment centers (your state)," "brain injury association (your state)" are limited only by your creativity. Typically, licensure agencies have mailing lists available—sometimes free of charge.

Usually, the staff at such centers are paraprofessionals who are highly qualified to assist clients in specific tasks, but mental health professionals from outside clinics often receive referrals for services such as counseling, group therapy, psychological evaluations, and consulting. Some centers routinely refer their clients to mental health professionals, and others may not be aware that such services could take place at their facility.

Ask the director of the facility if you can speak at a staff meeting to explain your services. When you speak to the group keep it brief, leave plenty of handouts, and try to be interesting and informative. Few mental health professionals extend the promotion of their services to this level.

When advertising to group homes and treatment centers emphasize that you take third-party payments (if you do). It is not likely that group homes or treatment centers will pay you out of their funds. They are typically a business, also, and are interested in making a profit, or at least breaking even. If you accept third-party payments you could actually save the treatment center money by providing a service for which they may not have to pay professional staff.

Example of the Potential Positive Effects of a Brochure

I once sent approximately 25 brochures to area CD treatment centers. Within a few weeks a large treatment center requested a psychological evaluation for a client. An appointment was made in less than 1 week (per clinic policy). Prior to meeting the client, time was spent with the director to determine specifically what they are looking for in an evaluation. The director suggested a specific outline, and then stated he was used to waiting at least a month or more for an evaluation, and two more weeks for the report. It was further noted that there had been several instances in which a client had been discharged before the center received the report.

The appointment was made within a few days of the referral and the report was sent to them within four days (per clinic policy). The report followed a format concordant with the director's request. Staff at the center said they were pleased, and that the report was helpful for treatment. Since that time (1997) the treatment center has referred clients solely to my practice.

In the rare instances clients from the treatment center do not have insurance, the evaluation is conducted pro bono. The combination of an informative brochure, service in a timely manner, and meeting the client's needs are the foundation for a successful practice. Do not be afraid to conduct free services at times. We are in the helping profession!

OTHER MENTAL HEALTH PROFESSIONALS

Referrals from other mental health professionals are most likely to take place if you practice in a specialty area. Generalists typically do not receive referrals from other therapists because they likely offer the same services the referral source offers. However, if you or others at your clinic have expertise in an area that is not offered by many others, the possibility of receiving referrals increases.

Receiving a referral from a fellow professional is an honor. It suggests that the referral source trusts your ability to provide services to their clients. There are at least five main points to remember when you receive referrals from fellow professionals: (a) reciprocate referrals, (b) coordinate insurance benefits with the referral source, (c) never steal a client, (d) always speak highly of the referral source to the client, and (e) send a letter of appreciation to the referral source.

Reciprocating Referrals

Receiving referrals is a give-and-take process. If you expect to receive referrals, plan on giving them as well. The referral process is symbiotic, each helps the other.

Since referrals generally come from professionals who do not provide the service requested, it is wise to find out what services they do provide in order to send them referrals for services you do not offer. If this scenario does not exist, do your best to reciprocate. Be sure to ask them what type of referrals they might be interested in receiving. Some clinics are so busy that they do not want additional referrals. Examples of referral reciprocation include:

Therapist 1	*Therapist 2*
Individual therapy for family members	Family therapy
Mental health treatment	Chemical dependencies
Psychological evaluations	Psychological therapy
Individual therapy	Group therapy
Adults in a family	Children in a family
Victim	Perpetrator

Coordinating Insurance Benefits

When a referral is made it is quite possible that both providers may work with the client simultaneously. Some insurance benefits limit the number of sessions per week, or only pay once per year for certain diagnostic services. If the two providers bill the insurance company, for example, in the same week for services that have time limits, only one provider will be paid. Always check with the insurance company about benefit limitations and discuss the situation with the other provider. If problems arise due to the insurance company declining to pay, it could result in both therapists losing the client, or termination of referrals from the referral source.

Never "Steal" a Client

When referrals are made it is extremely important for the two therapists to communicate which services are being referred. Sometimes, after a referral has been made, the referral source plans on never seeing the client again. At other times, the referral is intended to be temporary, such as when a specific service being conducted.

Sooner or later, you will receive a referral that was meant to be for a specific, temporary service, and the client will ask you to become his or her therapist. They will tell you how much more they

---

Example of a Poor Way of Starting a Private Practice

When you leave a clinic to start a private practice or join another clinic, you will be tempted to take clients with you. I recall an incident in the mid-1990s, in which a therapist worked in a large clinic and built up a large clientele within a few months. One day, he abruptly turned in his resignation. The clinic director then asked him about transferring his clients to other therapists within the clinic. The therapist stated that all of his clients were being discharged, and needed no more treatment.

It turned out that the therapist transferred his entire caseload to his new, private practice. He would now make a commission of 100 percent, instead of 50 percent. He believed that since he had a full caseload the practice would perpetuate itself due to referrals generated from his clients.

When he told his clients that his new office was located in his home about half of them went back to the previous clinic, stating that they felt uncomfortable going to the therapist's home for professional services. Almost all of his remaining clients eventually ended services within 2 months. Private practice was no longer what it seemed when he left his position. The practice soon closed.

Although it is not necessarily unethical to take clients with you, the long-term effect on your reputation can be marred if the process is not handled appropriately. Obtain consent from the previous employer and have valid reasons why certain clients would be better off remaining with you.

Lesson: Simply having a large client load does not make for a private practice. Clients expect a certain level of professionalism and many will not receive therapy in someone's home. Since most clients remain in treatment about six to ten sessions, a practice will not be viable very long without a means of receiving new referrals.

like you than the other therapist, and generally try to win you over. If you decide to become the client's primary therapist it will not only end a source of referrals, but it could damage your reputation among professionals if the referral source tells them what you did.

Always Speak Highly of the Referral Source to the Client

The referral source has sent you referrals because of a respect for the quality of work you conduct. When they send clients to you, reciprocate the respect. Never speak negatively to clients about the referral source. Chances are that if you do, referrals will cease. If clients speak negatively about the referral, do not add fuel to the fire. Of course, if a client talks about blatant ethical violations, you are required to investigate.

Send a Letter of Appreciation to the Referral Source

Always thank referral sources when you receive a referral. A signed, hand-written thank you card is suggested, because it shows that you personally filled it out and appreciate them sending you a client. Send a thank you note for every client, not simply at holiday times, or when you need more business. Few clinics follow this practice. It makes you stand out as someone who appreciates referral sources.

SCHOOLS

Some schools refer and others do not. Those that do not usually have a policy against it due to liability issues. Some schools do not give out specific referrals, but will provide a list of several mental health professionals that the client's parents may use to choose a provider. School referrals are generally due to behavior problems, ADHD, emotional problems, or family issues. School counselors, psychologists, and social workers typically have very busy schedules and may not have the time to conduct psychotherapy on a regular basis.

It can be somewhat difficult to work your way into a school system, because referrals come from a range of sources such as teachers, counselors, or principals. Advertising to schools generally works best by asking to attend a faculty meeting where all of these sources would be present. Some schools contract with therapists at the school board level.

MEDICAL PROFESSIONALS

As with schools, some medical professionals refer clients for counseling, while others tend to prescribe medications only. Usually, the best source of referrals comes from family practitioners. They are often the first medical professional to see a client, thus they are often the gatekeeper for referrals. Often, people with physical symptoms similar to mental health symptoms will first contact their primary physician, seeking a medical solution to their problems. This physician may or may not have sufficient training in mental health.

Physicians tend to be very busy and many do not have time for a meeting to discuss your services. A brief, professionally appealing flier sent out about every few months will likely increase your name recognition. Educational material that emphasizes the relationship between physical and psychological factors is helpful. When a referral is made find out if the physician desires brief progress reports, and what level communication is preferred. You may be asked to help evaluate the effects of medications being prescribed.

Some physicians will refer clients to you who habitually make medical appointments, but show few physical problems. Making psychological progress is usually quite difficult because of the client's low insight into the nature of his or her psychological concerns. However, being client centered and empathic may slowly bring about increased insight and change.

THE YELLOW PAGES

The effects of phone book advertising have changed since the onset of managed care. In the past clients often found local clinics by searching *The Yellow Pages*. Although this is still the case, there is an increasing trend for clients to check their provider manual, or contact their managed care customer service department and ask which clinics take their insurance.

In my experience, the number of referrals from phone book ads have decreased proportionately to the increase in referrals that originate from managed care. Even with the decrease in referrals *The Yellow Pages,* in most cases, is still a good source of referrals. However, clients tend to phone the largest ad, which may cost well over $1,000 per month in larger markets. The rates are negotiable. It is not uncommon for the company to agree to place an ad at the rate of the next smaller ad, or to ask for a three-color ad at the price of one color. Negotiate the price. Never pay the asking price for advertising.

When you sign up for a *Yellow Page*'s ad you commit yourself to 1 year of payments. If the payment is not made, your phone may get turned off. Thus, some advertisers add another phone line that is only published in *The Yellow Pages.* This serves two purposes: (a) You can directly track which referrals came from the ad, and (b) if for some reason the phone number is disconnected, or you decide to discontinue the ad, you still have your main phone line (as long as that number is not listed in your advertisement).

Most phone book markets offer a small, but free, listing in *The Yellow Pages.* You must contact them for this service. Of course, they will try to sell you an upgrade. Do not be afraid to make a very low offer, for the first year only, with the intent to see if this type of advertising is successful for you. As with brochures, do not write too much information in the ad or it will look too busy. Appeal to the client's needs, not just the virtues of the clinic. Most markets also offer Internet ads for a reasonable price.

THE INTERNET

Web pages are clearly a growing market. They provide an opportunity to present multifaceted information about the clinic, therapists, services, policies, and any other information you want to provide.

Two main issues are noted—the quality and accessibility of the Web site. Unless you are very experienced in Web page design, it is suggested to have this performed by a professional. They have the experience and know what works. Prices can range from a few hundred dollars to thousands, so be careful. There are predesigned Web sites available that allow you to fill information in various templates, and provide choice of graphics and typestyles. There is wide variation in quality when using templates. The other issue is accessibility. Use the rule, "The more accessible, the more expensive." You can pay various search engines increasing amounts to place your ad higher in the order of displayed Web sites. At the same time, do not make the keywords so general that too many people, not intending to view the site, will be directed toward it. This could be quite costly because prices are generally based on *hits,* or the number of times the site is visited. For example, if your site comes up with the keyword *psychology,* and the person clicks on your site, you will be charged even if that person's intent was simply to look for a psychology term.

Spend time thinking of keywords that increase the chances of potential clients viewing your site. Practice typing in keywords to see what comes up. A professional Web site designer will inform you of your various options.

MANAGED CARE AND INSURANCE COMPANIES

These can be an excellent source of referrals. You do not have to pay for advertising, postage, or travel. Many insurance clients contact their insurance provider's customer service or case management departments for referrals. These departments typically have a list of qualified providers organized by location and specialty. Keep in contact with the staff of insurance companies who make referrals. A few minutes spent introducing yourself on the phone and thanking them for each referral received leads to you standing out when they need someone with the services you provide. Just as in any business, public relations is a necessary skill.

PREVIOUS CLIENTS

Perhaps the greatest honor to a clinic is to generate referrals from previous clients. In larger, established clinics the greatest percentage of referrals is often from previous clients. There is no advertising expense when previous clients refer people to you.

If at all possible, try to match the client to the same therapist as the referral source. They will typically ask for this therapist by name. If that therapist is no longer at your clinic, offer them another option, but do not withhold the name of the clinic where the requested therapist is now working (unless the therapist requests you not to give out this information).

SUMMARY

Therapists who are business oriented and creative look for referral sources. They do not shy away from the business aspects of their position, because these aspects are their bread and butter. Because most therapists tend to not be business oriented, those who are willing to learn some basic skills are often able to expand their practice in a relatively brief period of time.

A lack of referral sources is akin to a store with plenty of merchandise but no customers. Simply waiting for referrals without putting in the legwork, public relations effort, and advertising is almost a guarantee of failure.

Clinic brochures can either be a gold mine or an unnecessary expense. A simple, colorful brochure that highlights the strengths of your clinic is likely to be read. A wordy, black-and-white brochure with no graphics is a waste of time and money. It portrays low-quality work.

When opening a new clinic follow The Golden Rule: Treat others how you would want them to treat you. Do not open a new clinic until you are financially ready, and are reasonably assured that you have a source of referrals. Leave your present position on good terms, ensuring your employer knows your plans. Do not take any of your client load and/or referral sources with you without the consent of your employer. Put yourself in the shoes of your employer, who likely went through much expense and time to obtain the referral sources and clients that you are seeing.

Clinicians who open a clinic by stealing clients have few business scruples. If they cannot operate with this basic level of respect for their previous employer, they are likely to have other business issues or ethical concerns. Few clinics who begin in this manner survive very long. Many therapists suffer from a poor reputation after making such a move.

Maintaining a balance between being a caring therapist and a businessperson is crucial. A therapist is always a therapist. Certain characteristics, such as having compassion for others and being a good listener and helper, are basic qualifications. A therapist going into business or directing a clinic remains a therapist, but also learns business principles so that the clinic can remain in operation.

Starting or managing a mental health practice solely for profit is not a good decision. There will be several times when decisions will be made to not charge clients, provide free services, and make choices that do not appear to be very business oriented.

TEST YOUR KNOWLEDGE

1. The most effective clinic brochures

    (a) contain a detailed list of each service the clinic provides.

    (b) provide a summary of services and are visually appealing.

    (c) must be printed professionally.

    (d) are black-and-white.

2. How frequently should advertising be sent out to the same recipients?

    (a) Weekly

    (b) Monthly

    (c) Never advertise more than once to the same place

    (d) Periodically, at a pace to keep up with referrals

3. If you receive a referral from a therapist to provide family counseling, and one of the family members asks you if you would

see a friend who needs counseling, what is the best practice to follow?

    (a) Refuse to see the client.

    (b) Discuss the issue with the original referral source.

    (c) Make an appointment.

    (d) Wait until the family counseling is finished.

4. A referred client tells you that you are a much better therapist than the referral source. What would be the best course of action?

    (a) Phone the referral source and tell them what the client said.

    (b) Consider reporting the problem to the licensure board.

    (c) Talk positively about the referral source.

    (d) Ignore what the client is saying.

5. A referral source has sent you multiple referrals. How might you show your appreciation in an ethical manner?

    (a) Send the referral source a check.

    (b) Send a thank you note.

    (c) Take him or her out to lunch.

    (d) Two of these.

Answers: 1. b; 2. d; 3. b; 4. c; 5. d

5

Hiring, Training, Paying, and Keeping Employees

The quality of any clinic is no higher or lower than the quality of its staff and management. A high level of professionalism, ethical behavior, accurate billing, documentation, and people skills is required to run a successful clinic. Therefore, do not rush into hiring new employees, and, when hired, let them know, up front, what level of performance is expected from them.

Clients expect much from the staff of a mental health clinic. They typically behave toward the staff as if they (the staff) were mental health professionals. Clients commonly attempt to discuss their issues with the receptionist or others working at the clinic. Although this level of trust may have merits, administrative staff must be carefully trained in how to redirect such conversations.

THE RELATIONSHIP WITH YOUR EMPLOYEES

It is possible that you will see your staff as much, or more, than your friends and loved ones. Decide up front what boundaries you will have in your work relationships. Because each employee has different needs in how they relate to their employer, problems can easily arise. Give employees no reason to believe that you have favorites or that you do not care for them. However, it may happen anyway based on their interpersonal needs and experiences.

Example of a Disgruntled Therapist

Several years ago I interviewed a therapist for employment. The pay for the position was based on a commission of collected funds, which is typical in many mental health clinics. During the interview, the applicant asked me what the average salary was of therapists who work at the clinic. I told her the average amount, and she accepted the position.

After a few months, the therapist quit and told me that she was going to sue me for everything I had because she was making less than the amount I had promised her. She referred to the average amount that other therapists made.

Actually, many therapists made much more income than the average amount, but part-timers made less. This therapist's average number of client visits was about three to four, then they terminated receiving services from her. Thus, there was less of an income compared to therapists who saw clients for more sessions. Even though the new therapist received an equal number of referrals within the clinic, her income was lower than most of the therapists, due to not keeping clients.

Over the next few months, after she left, she regularly phoned me demanding large sums of money and regularly threatened a lawsuit. Eventually, she stopped calling. No lawsuit was filed. She has worked at numerous clinics since that time, with an average stay of about 6 months.

Lesson: Be very clear when discussing issues such as salaries, benefits, advancement, and other areas with job applicants. Do not let applicants misconstrue general statements as promises. Carefully check their background and employment history. Therapists who have a history of working at clinics for no more than several months are more of a financial liability than an asset.

A manager's attitude is clearly reflected in staff morale. Some employees will attempt to be your close friend, while others keep a distance. Some employees respect, while others resent, authority. It is difficult to pick up on this during the initial interview because most people behave ideally in an interview situation. Even checking references may not be helpful.

Consistency is the key. Although it may be extremely difficult, be consistent across the board in your dealings with employees in areas such as income, job duties, advancement, time off, and other areas that can lead to perceived inequities. Have clearly written policies and procedures that apply to everyone. Go over employment policies and procedures with every newly hired person. After their staff training, obtain a signature verifying they have read and understand the clinic's policies and procedures. Even if you hire someone you have known for years, remain consistent, and subject everyone to the same policies.

Managerial inconsistency leads to disgruntled employees, resentment, poor work performance, and high turnover. Whenever it even appears that someone is receiving preferred treatment,

---

Example of Problems Arising When Employees Are Treated Differently

I once purchased and managed a clinic where a variety of commissions had been paid to different employees. And, as in many places of employment, most people knew how much others were compensated. It became apparent that not all therapists were treated equally in this matter.

For example, one therapist was paid 20 percent more commission than other therapists. The clinic actually lost money when she saw clients. When asked why she was paid more, she stated that several years ago there was sickness in her family, and she needed additional income to pay ongoing medical bills. At that time, the clinic management gave her a surprisingly high raise. A few months after I purchased the clinic, I asked how her family was doing. She stated that everything was fine. The problems that had required a higher pay rate no longer existed. Then, when the possibility of returning to a commission rate similar to what others were earning was discussed, she became upset, stating that the clinic could not legally lower her commission because she was under contract. As time went by, it became quite apparent that she did not follow several of the policies and procedures of the clinic and was a definite liability in a number of ways. It turned out that most of the other therapists knew that she was not working as hard, but was making more money, leading to resentment. When her contract was up for renewal she was offered a commission that was commensurate with the rest of the clinicians with similar experience. She then quit, and within about a week she contacted other therapists stating that I was going to lower their commission rates by 20 percent. That didn't happen.

Lesson: Do not give specific employees special treatment. Even if it is meant to be temporary, the employee will have difficulty giving up the special treatment. In addition, if other employees discover this action, they will feel shorted.

problems arise. Although the authoritarian employer who says, "I'm the boss. I make the decisions around here," may be technically correct, that philosophy usually leads to a stifling work environment. Most mental health workers prefer to be employed in a work environment that promotes a democratic decision-making process.

JOB DESCRIPTIONS

Every position in the clinic should have a well-defined job description. Specific and potential duties should be clearly listed. If an employee changes duties during the course of employment, rewrite the job description and obtain a signature. Job descriptions are typically not written for each employee or contractor, but for the specific job title. For example, if two administrative personnel have different duties, they should have different job descriptions and titles.

When writing job descriptions, include anything that could potentially be included in the job, and also include a statement that could cover out of the ordinary tasks in a statement such as, "and other duties assigned by the supervisor." If an employee's new tasks (other duties) become routine, amend the job description to specifically include these tasks.

Employers become weary of hearing the phrase, "That's not in my job description." Actually, they shouldn't assign tasks that are not in a job description. Therefore, think ahead when writing job descriptions, including items such as covering for vacant positions or when other employees are on leave or ill. Consider future plans for the business when additional duties might be needed.

Routinely ask employees about their duties and work environment. Periodically ask them if there have been any changes in their duties in order to revise their job description. An interested employer is much more likely to have workers who "go the extra mile" than a distant employer.

The main point is that job descriptions are for the benefit of both the employee and the employer. They are intended to adequately communicate what is expected in job duties.

Example of a Job Description for a Therapist in a Mental Health Clinic

Therapist Responsibilities

A. *Assessment*

   1. Completes a comprehensive assessment in a competent and timely manner (due by second session).

   2. Demonstrates a professional working knowledge of psychopathology, making an accurate diagnosis.

   3. Demonstrates knowledge of normal developmental milestones as they relate to mental illness and is able to differentiate a milestone versus a significant issue.

   4. Demonstrates a knowledge of chemical dependency as it relates to mental illness and has the ability to make a differential diagnosis.

   5. Can adequately provide a differential diagnosis in areas such as differentiating between Axis I and Axis II diagnoses.

B. *Treatment Planning*

   1. Completes the treatment plan by the completion of the second session.

   2. Completes the treatment plan in a competent manner.

   3. Creates a treatment plan containing behavioral goals and objectives.

   4. Completes status reviews in a timely manner (every 90 days).

   5. Creates status reviews that clearly document the course of treatment utilizing measurable objectives and a reasonable length of stay.

   6. Completes discharge summaries within 15 days of discharge.

   7. Engages with the client in aftercare planning and documents accordingly in the discharge summary.

C. *Case Management*

   1. Adheres to professional ethical standards during the case management.

   2. Has the ability to locate appropriate resources for the client as needed.

   3. Communicates with referral sources as needed.

   4. Seeks case consultation as needed.

   5. Obtains third party authorizations as needed.

   6. Makes appropriate referrals.

D. *Treatment Modalities*

1. Documents the appropriate type therapy as practiced (e.g., not documenting individual therapy if marital therapy is being conducted).

2. Has a professional knowledge of billable treatment modalities and seeks consultation when needed.

3. Provides services only in areas credentialed both by licensure board and the clinic.

4. Receives ongoing continuing education in areas of competency.

5. Maintains involvement in respective professional organizations.

E. *Clinic Involvement*

1. Attends and participates in monthly staff meetings.

2. Participates in process improvement groups or shows interest in improving the quality of care for clients and procedures.

3. Attends and participates in case consultations.

4. Shares knowledge and resources with other clinicians.

5. When experiencing a grievance, addresses the appropriate staff to resolve the problem.

6. Works cooperatively with other staff and supervisors.

F. *Additional Responsibilities*

1. Adheres to the contractual agreement in client productivity by seeing a minimum of ____ clients per month.

2. Follows policies and procedures for safety.

3. Demonstrates knowledge of safety drill procedures.

4. Demonstrates knowledge of policies concerning client rights and confidentiality.

5. Follows organizational policy and procedures of universal precautions.

*Example of a Job Description for Physician / Medical
Director in a Mental Health Clinic*

Physician Responsibility

The Center recognizes the importance of a multidisciplinary approach to treatment. Therefore, the following actions have been initiated to ensure physician involvement in all cases:

1. The physician will review and certify the initial evaluation, mental status exam, diagnosis, treatment plan, and therapist assignment of all cases.

2. The physician will also review clients' medical history to determine the need for further examination or evaluation and take appropriate action.

3. The physician will be responsible for all admissions and discharges.

4. The physician will review the treatment plan for accuracy, and to determine the need for ongoing treatment, and certify this through his or her signature on the treatment plan.

5. The physician will review and certify the appropriateness of continued treatment through the quarterly status review.

6. The physician will review the appropriateness of discharges and the discharge diagnosis and will certify this through his or her signature on the discharge summary form.

7. The physician will review the need for medication and then take appropriate action.

8. The physician will review the need for change in treatment level when the client fails to respond to the present treatment.

9. The physician may consult on health care issues that impact the well being of the client and that can be expected to impact the treatment of the client.

10. The physician may be asked to explain to the client treatment that is outside the therapist's area of expertise. The client has the right to have all treatment explained to them in a manner they can understand. If the client is unable to understand the nature of the treatment or if explaining the treatment is medically unadvisable, this information may be given to another person on the patient's behalf.

11. The patient has the right to refuse treatment to the extent permitted by law and to be informed of the medical consequences of this action. The physician may be asked to explain this action to the patient.

12. The physician is expected to insure that all medical treatments are administered in accordance with all accepted clinical practices.

13. The physician is responsible to review the informed consent form with a patient who has been prescribed a medication to ensure that the patient has a full understanding of the benefits and risks associated with the medication. This will be documented by the patient's and physician's signature on the informed consent form.

14. The physician reports to the medical director for supervision, clarification of duties, job performance evaluations, and other aspects of job requirements.

Example of a Job Description for Office Support Staff in a Mental Health Clinic

Office Support Staff Responsibility

A. *General Office Duties*

1. Answer telephone (e.g., timely response, take messages accurately and appropriately, or place the call into voice mail system or transfer calls).

2. Greet clients.

3. Process new clients (e.g., offer and explain paperwork; verify completion, signature, and consents; obtain insurance information; and input face sheets).

4. Schedule psychiatric appointments.

5. Triage psychiatric calls.

6. Monitor mail (e.g., stamp, send, and distribute; make address corrections, follow up with return mail).

7. Update client information on computer system as needed.

8. Prepare client charts.

9. Refill clinical and office form bins.

10. Appropriately distribute contents of front office bins (e.g., fee agreements, transcription).

11. Fax and distribute faxes.

12. Attend office staff meetings.

13. Participate in process improvement group meetings as needed.

14. Complete staff correspondence.

B. *Facility-Related Duties*

1. Monitor kitchen (e.g., clean, refill supplies, make coffee).

2. Monitor and ensure cleanliness of common areas, group therapy rooms, and play room areas.

3. On Friday, polish waiting room furniture and dust office furniture, and multipurpose room.

C. *Payment- and Billing-Related Duties*

1. Verify all charge journals are correct and turned in, using appointment books for information.

2. Enter charges daily into billing system.

3. Update client information on the billing system.

4. Assist in processing insurance rejections and follow-ups, as requested by billing manager.

5. Print patient hard copies, as requested.

6. Request payments from clients.

7. Verify the accuracy of payments to be made (e.g., correct co-pay amount, check outstanding balances, check collection status).

8. Write receipts and give to clients.

9. Thoroughly complete and receipt journal for each transaction.

10. Flag problem accounts.

11. Correspond with billing department as needed.

12. Answer clients' billing questions.

13. Explain and witness fee agreement forms.

14. Enter client diagnosis on the computer system and follow up as needed.

D. *Opening- and Closing-Related Duties*

1. Balance payment information and distribute documents or information appropriately.

2. Place voice mail system on nighttime mode at the end of the day.

3. Turn on or off appropriate lights.

4. Lock and unlock specific areas of the clinic.

5. Computer system log off.

6. Secure and maintain cash drawer.

7. Turn on or off specific electronic equipment.

E. *Performance Improvement Responsibilities*

1. Demonstrate knowledge of performance improvement process.

2. Understand and follow policies and procedures.

3. Understand and follow safety policies and procedures.

4. Demonstrate knowledge of role in fire drills and other disaster procedures.

5. Follow organizational policies and procedures concerning the use of universal precautions.

6. Maintain current CPR certification, if appropriate.

7. Demonstrate knowledge of policies concerning client rights and confidentiality.

8. Demonstrate knowledge of policies regarding organizational ethics and acts in an ethical manner.

THERAPISTS—CONTRACT VERSUS EMPLOYEE

In most private practice situations, management must decide if therapists hired are going to be employees or independent contractors. Employees are on the regular payroll and are paid either a salary, hourly pay, or a commission. Most employees, if full time, are paid a salary. They are expected to see a certain number of clients per week and have other assigned tasks such as serving on committees, being on a rotation for emergency calls, supervising interns, and working on new referral sources. Typical employee taxes are deducted from their paychecks, and they may receive benefits such as insurance, vacation time, and retirement.

Contracted workers may work at the clinic, but not directly for the clinic. They are not paid benefits, and income taxes are not taken from their paycheck. They sign a contract that depicts their duties, responsibilities, relationship to the clinic, and payment. It is most common for contracted workers to be paid a commission on funds received. Financial and administrative arrangements for contracted workers vary significantly. In some clinics, they must do their own billing and schedule their own appointments. Sometimes they pay for office space and clerical help.

The IRS carefully scrutinizes the contractual relationship. When a contracted worker has a designated office, a business card with the name of the clinic, regular office hours, their name on company letterhead, a fairly long standing and continuous relationship with the clinic, and meets other conditions that fail to distinguish the contractor from an employee relationship, the IRS may deem this person as an employee and subsequently require the clinic to pay the employer's portion of back taxes (which could be a substantial amount).

The positive aspects of being an employee are job security, benefits, a stable salary, and not having to file self-employment tax information. The positive aspects of being an independent contractor are being able to deduct more business expenses when filing taxes, usually having a higher paycheck, and having a sense of independence. At this time, independent contractors typically receive anywhere from 35 to 80 percent of funds collected. The average is about 50 to 55 percent. If a clinic pays contracted employees over 60 percent, they will likely not make a profit. One of the major reasons so many private practices go out of business is from paying too high of a commission to professional staff.

SCREENING EMPLOYEES

Effective employee screening is crucial, especially in the mental health field. It is important to check references and document what they say about the employee. There are at least three types of possible references you can inquire into: personal (friends, acquaintances), professional (teachers, colleagues), and previous employers. Ask references very specific questions. Taken together, each of these sources can provide you with an accurate perspective of the applicant. Always conduct a criminal background check and, after hiring, repeat the procedure yearly. Be aware of the laws regarding what information can and cannot be collected in an interview to avoid any suggestion of discrimination.

During the interview process, do not make one person solely responsible for interviewing and hiring applicants. Interviews with different personnel, in both group and individual settings, will help provide the clinic with more than one perspective of the applicant's strengths and weaknesses. Considering that the applicant could be with the clinic for years and will affect fellow employees either positively or negatively, much time and consideration is needed before making a hiring decision.

Therapists

If the applicant is applying for a therapy position, ask very specific questions regarding why they left their previous positions (e.g., quit, fired, laid off). Always check for any negative history with clients, such as sexual or financial misconduct, harassment, or any other type of complaint. Contact their licensure board to determine if there have been any complaints, suspensions, or other disciplinary actions. Inquire whether any malpractice claims have been filed. Some states require that you check with every previous employer about any history of sexual misconduct. If the previous employer does not respond, and subsequent sexual misconduct occurs at your workplace, that employer could share part of the liability if an incident takes place. Or, if you hire someone with a known history of sexual misconduct, your clinic could share the liability if an offense occurs. Therefore, clearly document the steps you take to determine any history of sexual misconduct or any other potential problem areas.

Ask applicants to provide specific evidence (i.e., training, experience, supervision) of their specialties, clientele, therapeutic stance, and other areas of importance to your clinic. Beware of the therapist who says, "I see all ages and diagnoses of clients." Perhaps this might work with clients who have minor adjustment issues, but treatment for chronic mental health problems is highly specialized. For example, symptoms of Borderline Personality Disorder and Bipolar II can be very similar, but they are treated quite differently, and generic counseling will likely be unhelpful to either client. Therefore, spend an ample amount of interviewing time evaluating the therapist's expertise. Remember, it is considered malpractice to treat a client if you do not have sufficient training, supervision, and experience in their problem area.

You wouldn't ask a medical general practitioner to perform a heart transplant. Although mental health treatment is not as sophisticated as this example, the underlying principle holds true. When you interview a therapist who describes working in a specialty area, be sure to ask "heart transplant" questions, not general practitioner questions. This person will represent your clinic, so be thorough. If the applicant knows the material well, he or she will be impressed, rather than upset, with your questions.

Interviews and background checks are very important aspects of hiring therapists, but more information is needed to make an informed decision. Ask for work samples such as name-deleted reports, intakes, treatment plans, and progress notes. When you look at documentation such as treatment plans, ask them to explain how the plan relates to the diagnosis and subsequent treatment. Such questions are not designed to embarrass the applicant, but it helps you decide how much training will be necessary if the applicant is hired.

Example of Providing a Thorough Interview before Hiring a Therapist

I once sought to hire a child psychologist to direct a child psychology program. One applicant went through two interviews with other therapists in the clinic before the final interview, which I conducted. The previous interviews provided positive feedback about the applicant's personality, enthusiasm, and reference checks.

When questions were asked about the specialty of child psychology, the applicant discussed various experiences counseling children. Most of the responses were brief and general. It turned out that the applicant did not specialize in child psychology, but simply enjoyed counseling children. His internship was at a college counseling center, and his subsequent experience was in a few general private practices. The applicant was hired, not as the director of the program, but as a therapist who would receive adequate supervision and training to add a child psychology specialty to his credentials. Training and experience, not desire, lead to credentials.

Some Possible Interview Questions for Therapist Include the Following:

1. Tell me about yourself.
2. What is it about this clinic that led you to apply for the position?
3. What is your specialty?
4. What are your favorite and least favorite client problem areas to work with?
5. Which age groups do you see?
6. Are there any client groups you are not willing to see? Why not?
7. What is the average number of sessions you see a client?
8. How many clients do you typically see per day?
9. What theoretical stance do you incorporate into therapy? Why?
10. What do you like most and least about being a therapist?
11. What do you think causes people to change in therapy?
12. What is the most common reason clients terminate therapy with you?
13. Why did you leave or why are you leaving your last position?
14. What is your most common reason for leaving an employment position?
15. What are you looking for in this position?
16. What do you see yourself doing in 5 years? 10 years?
17. What are your continuing education plans?
18. What type of supervision do you prefer?
19. What are your greatest strengths and weaknesses?
20. What do you expect from your employer?
21. What days and hours are you willing to work?
22. What are your expectations for compensation?
23. In what ways would you be an asset to this clinic?
24. What would you do in the following clinical situation? (Describe an ambiguous scenario with an ethical dilemma.)
25. What questions do you have?

During the interview, assess their people skills and ability to respond to ambiguous questions. Their responses will likely be indicative of such skills in a counseling setting. For example, a person who is a good listener during the interview will likely be a good listener in therapy. His or her observed level of comfort in the interview may reflect how he or she acts with clients. The person's basic personality will change little from an interview to a counseling situation. Ask yourself, "Do I want this person to represent our clinic?"

If there appear to be some shortfalls, ask yourself if the person is trainable or seems willing to learn. Sometimes you have to go with your gut feelings about someone in an interview. He or she can be hired on a trial basis.

After the therapist is hired, set up at least a few days of orientation. This typically involves spending 2 to 4 hours with each department (e.g., billing, administrative, medical records, other therapists, clinical supervisors) in the clinic to learn how the clinic operates, and its policies and procedures. A well-managed clinic will have standard written policies and procedures in all areas of its operations. As in any business, any deviation can have a ripple effect. For example, if each therapist has a different way of organizing charts, billing clients, writing treatment plans, and so on, the result will be chaos. When a clinical supervisor or an auditor reviews a chart, it is expected that it follows the same format as other charts in the clinic. Standardization always leads to simplicity and efficiency.

An audit by an insurance company or an accrediting agency will be much smoother if each chart is organized the same. That is, when the chart is opened, the reviewer knows exactly where to find any needed information. For example, if the file has a center divider, there are four possible divisions for organizing files. They can be organized as follows (or any consistent format):

Section 1:   Demographic, financial, and background information; medical records.

Section 2:   Intake material, treatment plan and revisions.

Section 3:   Progress notes, discharge or termination papers.

Section 4:   Testing.

Provide each therapist with a policies and procedures handbook for areas that involve their position. This folder includes examples of what is expected concerning clinical forms, billing sheets, intake material, treatment plans, progress notes, discharge summaries, and so on. New therapists should be well-informed of how their work will be evaluated and what is expected from them. Overtraining is better than undertraining. If possible, have a system of mentor therapists to assist new therapists as they transition to the position.

Be acutely aware of the new therapist's background and attitude toward policies, procedures, documentation, and working in a standardized system. Maverick therapists tend to be a financial liability.

Managing a mental health clinic involves much more than just being able to consult with therapists in clinical matters. Performing in a management role adds a dimension of fiscal, legal, clinic growth, and supervisory responsibilities to your platter. It can be very difficult to transition from being a colleague or peer to other therapists, to being in a position requiring hiring, firing, and making fiscal decisions. The manager's first business responsibility is to keep the clinic afloat. At times this duty requires ending the employment of therapists who are well-liked by others in the clinic, but who are a liability in other ways. It is especially difficult when their fellow therapists do not know what led to the firing—and if you tell them you may be liable for slander. Thus, be careful who you hire.

The therapist who sees the most clients may not necessarily be the most profitable employee to the clinic. Attempt to hire therapists who are team oriented, care about their clients, abide by the policies and procedures of the clinic, practice within their competencies, are not prima donnas, and find creative means to improve the clinic's policies and services.

It does not take much time to fully appreciate the saying, "It is lonely at the top." In any group of people there will be leaders, followers, backers, complainers, mavericks, conformists, and much more. Every person is obviously entitled to his or her personality, but a good clinic manager will make all efforts to find the positive side of people and incorporate their strengths. However, when some

*Example of the Need for a Clinic to Train
and Monitor Therapists' Documentation*

I managed a clinic that received regular insurance audits due to a large volume of business. One of the employees was a well-liked and excellent therapist. However, he was usually behind in his paperwork, and he provided minimal documentation to verify the medical necessity of services. Whatever paperwork he did complete clearly did not match the protocol for the clinic. He stated that therapists should have the freedom to document items how they choose. Although the therapist was advised a number of times about his documentation procedures, he did not comply, eventually left the clinic, and started a cash-only practice.

Several months later, an insurance company conducted a periodic audit. They reviewed a set number of files from each therapist. Most of the files were well-documented, and no paybacks to the insurance company were necessary. However, this therapist's charts were poorly documented, and the insurance company demanded a few thousand dollars to be repaid. In other words, there was insufficient written evidence that the services provided were necessary and little documentation as to what took place in the sessions.

Even though the therapist had left the clinic, a bill was sent to him for the payback. He refused to pay, stating that he was never taught how to document what was required by the insurance company. Fortunately for the clinic, there were papers signed by the therapist verifying he received the appropriate training in his clinic orientation, attendance records from staff training, plus the therapist's contract stated that any paybacks to third-party payers are the responsibility of the therapist, not the clinic (for the amount of commissions received by the therapist).

Lesson: Being an effective therapist requires much more than providing therapy. Skills such as documentation are a must in this age of accountability. Without these skills, a therapist could place him- or herself or the clinic in financial trouble.

employees cannot or will not function in the best interest of the clinic, it is your job to manage them. Decisions can be very difficult, and feelings will often be hurt because of your decisions. Problems with therapists or any other employees should be taken care of immediately and require assertiveness.

Receptionists

Chapter 1 of this text discusses the benefits of a good receptionist. Hiring a receptionist should involve as much time and effort as hiring a therapist. The receptionist is the first person clients talk to on the phone and is the first person to greet the clients when they come to the clinic. Two main skills are needed: customer service abilities and organizational skills. The receptionist is clearly one of the most crucial staff members in a mental health clinic.

BILLING—IN-HOUSE VERSUS OUTSIDE BILLING

In the growth of a typical clinic, the therapist usually begins as a solo practitioner and fills out the billing forms at the end of each day. As the practice grows, there is little time available to check insurance benefits, obtain authorizations, bill, rebill, and perform the follow-ups required. Unless the therapist is doing quite well financially, it is not feasible to hire a biller in a small practice. As the practice grows, two options become available: hire a biller or utilize a billing service. Typically, the transition step is training the receptionist to do the billing. This practice usually works fairly well until the practice has grown too much.

Most mental health clinics are able to provide in-house billing if staff are adequately trained. Billing is a very complex job that requires many billing codes, rules, and regulations to be followed closely. Minor errors lead to rejections of payment by the insurance company. Many times, when a bill has been rejected, it is difficult to ascertain exactly why it was rejected and requires much time to straighten out. Thus, the transition from having a receptionist or therapist conduct the billing is a difficult time for most clinics.

An alternative is to use a service that specializes in mental health billing. Some services charge by the hour, some charge a percentage of the amount billed, some charge by the number of bills sent, and others charge a percent of funds received. This is usually negotiable. The key is to provide the biller with the correct information. Rebilling can take as much time as the initial billing, so if you make an error in the billing and it must be rebilled, expect to pay the fee twice if your arrangement is per bill or by the hour.

As a clinic grows, there will be a point where it becomes afford-able to hire a full-time or part-time biller, rather than use a billing service. A person working part time in billing could be a full-time employee in another capacity, such as scheduling or keeping med-ical records. Large clinics (30 or more therapists) generally have a full-time person in each of these positions.

THE BILLING PERSON

Whoever does your billing (yourself, clerical staff, billing depart-ment, or a professional biller), the process of billing is not simply submitting the invoice for services. The knowledge, clerical accu-racy, and persistence of the biller can have a dramatic effect on the amount collected.

Knowledge

Anyone can fill out the blank lines in an insurance form. But the idiosyncrasies and diverse policies of various insurance companies require learning the specific requirements for each. Although pro-cedures have become more standardized, the biller cannot assume one will be the same as others.

Make a list of billing requirements for each third-party payer. This list should include the following information:

1. Requirements for approval for services.
2. Number of services allowed without additional authori-zation.
3. Covered and noncovered services (e.g., testing, individual, group, family).
4. Covered and noncovered diagnoses.
5. Specific billing codes allowed and not allowed.
6. Time designations (e.g., 15, 30, 60 minutes) per unit of each billing code.

7. Number of services or units allowed per billing code.

8. Minimum time between services (billing codes).

9. What specific client information is required.

10. Deductible and co-payment amounts.

11. What benefits or number of services have already been used this year.

12. How to designate billing for supervisees, if covered.

Clerical Accuracy

The person who types the insurance information into the billing program must not make clerical errors. Mistakes such as typographical errors, incomplete information, items written on the wrong line, or any other incorrect information will likely result in a rejection of the claim. When claims are rejected, it may take more time to figure out the problem and resubmit the claim than filing the original. If the biller is paid by the hour, much time and money are wasted due to clerical inaccuracy in billing.

If your billing claims are often rejected by third-party payers, carefully investigate the source of the clerical problems that lead to the rejections. Sources of error could be in the administrative personnel who record insurance information, the therapist's log of services, the information sheet provided to the biller, or the biller's transposition of the information to the billing program. This information is not difficult to detect. When the source(s) of the billing errors is detected, provide education to your employees. If the concerns are with an outside billing service, decisions must be made whether you will continue its services.

Persistence

Too many therapists and clinics do not rebill an insurance company when payment is not received. This may be due to the nature of therapists, lack of business training, or lack of billing knowledge.

When a billing invoice is rejected, never assume that it will not be paid eventually. Carefully check the reason for the rejection. Clerical inaccuracies are easily corrected. Errors involving procedural concerns (see list in preceding section) may be more difficult to re-bill when a third-party billing procedure has not been followed.

Unless there is a blatant reason for a billing rejection, it is worthwhile to contact the third-party payer and discuss the reason for the rejection. Many times the rejection is made due to a misunderstanding, and the person representing the payer will instruct you how to rebill the claim. Persist in rebilling rejections until you are convinced that you should not be paid. For example, if a client has not paid an insurance deductible, you will not be paid by the insurance company for sessions corresponding to this amount. Or, if you provide two individual sessions in less than a week period and the insurance provisions allow no more than one session per week, you will not be paid unless there was a prior authorization for the extra service. As mentioned previously, it is very important to know the policies of every third-party payer for whom you are a provider.

When a billing department gives up too easily, the financial status of the clinic and therapists may be in jeopardy. Therefore, be persistent and assertive when dealing with third-party payers.

A common concern in many clinics is neglecting to collect insurance deductibles and co-payments from clients. Therapists often believe that clients who are going through emotional problems are not able to handle the added stress of paying a few hundred dollars in deductibles. If the average number of sessions clients are seen by a therapist is about six to ten and the deductible is waived, many problems exist. First, the therapist is in jeopardy of losing the contract with the payer. Second, if the deductible is $200, for example, about a quarter of the sessions will be for free, resulting in a significant financial loss if this procedure is followed for several clients.

SUMMARY

The personnel you hire could make or break your clinic; therefore, be very patient. Conduct a thorough background check. Be sure that the applicant's statements match their training and experience. Allow others to interview the applicant. Provide ample time to train the therapist in the policies and procedures of the clinic. If these procedures are followed, the clinic has a much higher chance of finding success with the new therapist.

When a clinic hastily hires a new therapist because it must fill a vacancy immediately, success is hit or miss. The clinic could set itself up for legal, ethical, therapeutic, financial, or an array of other potential problems that could have been screened and prevented if given enough time in the initial interview process.

Have specific policies and procedures that provide for equal treatment of employees. Do not have special employees who have different privileges than others. Such a system only promotes dissent and turnover. People will respect your fairness. Allow employees to be creative, and encourage them to be part of the team. Listen to their suggestions. Well-treated employees discover a sense of purpose and enjoy their job.

A clinic that has no specific policies and procedures will have personnel, clinical, and administrative problems. Although creativity should be rewarded, if it is not given parameters it can create chaos.

Both staff and therapists should be paid a fair and competitive wage. The amount of the wage is a balance between what will motivate the employee to remain on the job and what is necessary for the clinic to make a reasonable profit. When both the clinic and employees' financial needs are met, each is more prepared to help take care of clients' needs.

When employee compensation is too high, the clinic is at risk of becoming insolvent. When employee compensation is too low, there is usually a high staff turnover. Once an employee or contractor is overpaid, it is very difficult to lower wages when the clinic is in financial difficulty.

Billing is a necessary expense in a mental health clinic. Errors lead to nonpayment, thus sufficient time and effort is required. When the billing person in a clinic, or the billing service used, is efficient and knowledgeable, the maximum amount of the fee can be collected, and both the therapists and clinic benefit.

Some therapists seem to be afraid of asking clients for money.

They do not collect co-payments and deductibles, and do not pursue rejected claims. When therapists paychecks are low and the clinic makes little or no profit, everyone suffers.

TEST YOUR KNOWLEDGE

1. Written job descriptions are helpful because they
   (a) spell out exactly what employees are allowed to do.
   (b) motivate people to take on more responsibilities.
   (c) increase communication regarding duties between staff and management.
   (d) provide a basis for comparing employee's contributions to the company.

2. Which staff member is least apt to receive health insurance benefits from an employer?
   (a) Management
   (b) Clerical staff
   (c) Contracted therapists
   (d) Salaried therapists

3. What are the advantages of a small clinic using a billing service?
   (a) It might not be able to afford a biller.
   (b) The current employees may not be aware of billing procedures.
   (c) A billing service is trained in the intricacies of billing.
   (d) All of these.

4. If you hire a therapist you have not investigated and the therapist behaves in an inappropriate manner at your clinic, what might the consequences be to your clinic?
   (a) None, because a clinic is not responsible for the behavior of therapists.

(b) The clinic could be partially liable for what took place.

(c) The clinic is only responsible if the therapist is a salaried employee.

(d) The clinic has some responsibility only if it knew of the previous offenses.

Answers: 1. c; 2. c; 3. d; 4. b

6

Developing a Positive Professional Reputation

A positive reputation must be earned through hard work, high ethical standards, and professional competence. The media is all too quick to report the misdeeds of professionals. One gross error in judgment or an ethical mistake can collapse the career of a mental health professional. However, it takes years of consistency and excellent work to develop a positive reputation. The media does not seek out stories about therapists who behave ethically; this behavior is expected.

Both major and minor acts can help build one's reputation. Major acts tend to accelerate growth. Minor acts are more cumulative, but eventually produce the same result. The following list notes behaviors that can result in either a negative or positive reputation.

SEMINARS TO PROFESSIONALS

Seminars are an excellent method to both generate income and develop a professional reputation. You do not have to search for a seminar company to hire you. Anyone can perform the few tasks it takes to set up a seminar. The most difficult part is being an expert in a given area, having a topic that is of current interest, and getting people to attend the function. This information is based on over 200

Sure Reputation Wreckers	*Sure Reputation Builders*
Major concerns	
Excessive/improper billing	Conservative billing procedures
Clinical incompetence/malpractice	Clinical competency
Ethics violations	Strong and consistent ethical code
Smaller concerns	
Lengthy waiting lists	Prompt appointments
Habitually late starting times	Prompt starting times
Late reports	Prompt reports
Nonchalant demeanor	Professional/cordial demeanor
Self-aggrandizement (know it all)	Humility (lifelong learner)
Ignoring complaints	Quick response to complaints
Constant complainer	Listens and tries to better the situation
Charge money for everything	Volunteer some services
Tooting your own horn	Letting others toot the horn for you

Example of a Ruined Reputation

A struggling, but hardworking psychologist worked to build up a private practice in a metropolitan area. After about 10 to 15 years, the practice grew to a large, well-known mental health clinic. As he became more successful, he purchased more elaborate homes and cars. He spent more on vacations and many other luxuries that he could now afford before he became successful. He believed that he earned his new lifestyle and should be rewarded for his hard work.

One of his largest contracts involved a government organization that paid him directly for mental health services, rather than using the clients' insurance. The amount that the government agency paid was modest, and eventually he began to feel shorted by the level of payment. That is, he felt a psychologist as successful as himself should be paid more.

Many of these clients automatically gave him their insurance cards when they received services from him. He did not take the cards and told the clients that services were paid by the government agency, not their insurance company. As time went by, as in any business, there were ups and downs in the clinic's income; however, his spending habits increased, not allowing for the leaner times. After becoming increasingly more disgruntled about the fee he was paid, he rationalized that the government payment was like a coinsurance, paying only part of what was due to him. Gradually, he began billing the insurance companies of the clients who presented their insurance cards to him. In time, this led to asking most clients for their insurance cards and also billing their insurance.

Eventually, one of the clients who was aware that the government agency paid for services reported him to the government agency and to the board of psychology. The psychologist's fraudulent billing was in the newspaper from the time of the initial charges to the end of the legal proceedings.

He rationalized that his usual and customary fee was twice the amount that the agency paid, so he was simply billing the client's insurance for the other half. However, his contract with the government agency clearly stipulated that he could not charge the client or the client's insurance company for services. Insurance fraud clearly took place. Furthermore, he never noted that there was another payer on the claims to the insurance companies. The psychologist was convicted of insurance fraud, and his license to practice was revoked. He was required to pay back several thousand dollars to the insurance companies.

Lesson: Any of us can start out with noble intentions. As we become more established, we must not let greed get in the way of success, or it could result in a downfall. Define your success in terms of personal satisfaction and helping others. Don't allow money and possessions to be the measuring stick of your success, or you could become dependent on them for personal validation. Also, it can lead to rationalizing unethical practices you would not have considered previously.

seminars I have conducted nationally. I have learned as much information concerning what not to do as what to do.

The Following Steps are Suggested to Arrange and Conduct a Seminar

The Topic

You must be a well-experienced expert or at least very knowledgeable in a topic area that will draw interest from the audience you intend to address. Topics such as "Individual Therapy" or "Working with Adults" are much too vague and a part of the typical training

Example of This Writer's Seminar Experience

Soon after finishing graduate school, I began to notice that there was little consistency in paperwork and documentation at mental health clinics. My initial concerns were with documentation, due to an audit early in my career. I found that good documentation requires appropriate paperwork and forms.

Over a few years, I researched the forms used in several clinics and compared them to what information was requested by managed care, insurance companies, and accrediting agencies. Some forms were on target, while others completely missed the boat. As I put more forms together, more clinicians asked me for copies and to conduct staff training in documentation.

A friend of mine suggested conducting a local seminar. I purchased a mailing list and advertised a seminar in documentation. The attendance was surprisingly high, leading to more seminars. When I presented the seminars, I often referred to how the quality of the forms and paperwork can affect documentation. I suggested means of streamlining the process that actually took less time but collected more information. Then clinicians asked if they could purchase my forms.

I put together a packet of forms that sold tremendously well. This led to discussions with the publisher, John Wiley & Sons. I sent them a packet of forms and a copy of the handouts from my seminar on documentation. The result was the publishing of my first two books: *The Clinical Documentation Sourcebook,* a book of forms; and *The Psychotherapy Documentation Primer,* which trains clinicians in documentation procedures. Because of the popularity of the books, I have received several requests for seminars and staff trainings.

Lesson: If you see a need in the field, study it well. You will become an expert.

for mental health professionals—not seminar material. However, specific topics that meet either the therapeutic or professional needs of the intended audience are much more likely to attract interest. Some states have specific continuing education requirements, such as a certain number of hours spent each year in ethical, therapeutic, or other training. The key is to find the need and the potential drawing power of various topics.

Approval for Continuing Education

If your seminar is intended to provide required continuing education for fellow professionals, approval must be obtained from various mental health organizations. The approval process varies state by state. In some areas the licensure boards (e.g., psychology, social work, professional counseling, marriage and family) approve seminars for credit. Some approvals are through state professional organizations, while others are approved through national organizations (e.g., American Psychological Association, National Association of Social Workers). Some professional boards list qualifications for continuing education and simply require that their criteria are met.

Thus, it is very important to contact every mental health licensing organization in each state you are conducting seminars and specifically ask them for the requirements to be a continuing education (CE) provider. There is typically an approval fee, which is usually based on the number of hours the seminar lasts. Some organizations have a fee and charge you an amount of money for each participant who is receiving approval from them.

Try not to advertise a seminar before you receive CE approval. If you must, state that the approvals are pending. It takes about 2 to 6 weeks to receive an approval. Therefore, plan on conducting the seminar several weeks in advance, but do not spend too much money on it until you receive the CE approvals. The fliers you send out should tell which approvals have been secured. If you make a statement in your flier that approval is pending, be sure to provide a way to determine if it has been approved. If people preregister and the seminar is not approved, offer a full refund or admission to the next seminar at a reduced rate.

Location of the Seminar

The most common choices are hotel banquet rooms, college auditoriums, and lodging facilities with banqueting services available. The best location has the following characteristics: (a) convenient for driving, (b) low- or no-cost parking, (c) near an airport (for national seminars), (d) convenient lodging in a safe section of town, (e) convenient and quality dining near, but preferably at, the location; and (f) a moderate to upscale atmosphere.

Facilities at the Seminar Location

The following amenities are suggested. Be sure that the facility has (a) adequate audio-visual equipment, (b) comfortable and roomy seating, (c) privacy, (d) comfortable temperature control, (e) quality food service, and (f) sound containment.

Negotiating the Cost of the Facilities

If you are using a hotel, the most common setting for seminars, be prepared to negotiate. It is the job of hotel management to make the most profit as possible. The more profit they make, the less profit for you. If you do not negotiate, you could end up paying a few thousand dollars more than necessary. I have secured a number of very fine hotel banquet rooms at no charge when the initial asking price was up to $1,500.

The following procedure will help you negotiate the best rate. Using a professional letterhead, write or fax a letter to several high quality hotels in the area you desire to hold the seminar. Begin the letter with a paragraph describing that you conduct seminars for mental health professionals in various cities. Explain that you will be conducting a seminar in the area and are looking for a facility to fit your needs. Then let them know your company policy is to have the hotel cater the snacks and the meal for the seminar. Tell them that your budget for coffee, water, soft drinks, a morning snack, lunch, and an afternoon snack is, for example, $20 per person. Include the date, starting and ending times, estimated number of people, and what services are desired. Include a notation that the banquet room (seminar room) will be free of charge and the hotel room for the speaker is free for one night. The hotel is likely to accept these conditions if the guaranteed number of participants is over 100 participants. The average number of participants at seminars I conduct is usually about 125 to 140. If 100 people attend a seminar and the hotel receives $25 per person for the use of the room and food, the hotel intake, before expenses, is $2,500. Plus, if only 25 percent of the participants stay in the hotel overnight and the room charge is, for example, $80, the gross intake would include an additional $2,000. Thus, if the hotel allows you to use a banquet or seminar room for 8 hours, they could take in at least $4,500, less expenses. You are much more likely to receive the room for free if they have no other reservations on the day you requested. Therefore, make the proposal to several hotels.

When you set the price for the seminar, do not say that there is a $25 charge for refreshments and lunch, but, rather, advertise that lunch and refreshments are free of charge. Simply add $25 to your intended price of the seminar. Adding $25 to the price of a seminar should not affect attendance if the seminar topic is appealing. I have experimented with seminar prices in the past, and it made no difference in attendance if a seminar cost $79 or $139! Actually, people might not expect much from a bargain-priced seminar. If you charge a high price, be sure that they get their money's worth.

When contacting hotels, do not ask for their rates or for a bid. If you do, they will likely give you a fairly high quote. Typically, about 25 to 50 percent of the hotels you contact will respond to you when you present your budget and terms to them. Some will offer different terms, and some will accept your proposal. If you and a hotel agree on terms, be careful to have a clause that protects you if you must cancel the seminar. For example, if the seminar is on July 1, include a clause that you may cancel by June 10. Without a cancellation clause, you may be liable for any money the hotel would have received. It is likely that the hotel will want you to guarantee a certain number of participants. Keep the number as low as possible. If the number of participants who attend the seminar is lower than guaranteed, have a clause in the contract that stipulates how much money must be paid per the number of people below the guaranteed number. Be sure that your seminar registration deadline is at least a week before the cancellation date for the hotel. This will give you ample time to decide if the seminar will be profitable or if it should be cancelled.

If possible, reserve a room that will hold at least 25 percent more than your anticipated number of people. Often walk-ins come to the seminar. You can always add more tables and chairs if the room is large enough, but you cannot move walls if the room is too small.

When two or more hotels make you an offer, do not be afraid to ask competitors to beat each other's prices. Such a practice is common in business and is not insulting. Whenever you are negotiating or bargaining, be sure not to sacrifice quality. That is, do not provide a low quality meal or skimp on the refreshments. Participants are quick to complain when they pay over $100 for a seminar and are fed an unappetizing meal. Be sure that there are meal choices, including vegetarian options.

Paying for Help

If you are conducting a seminar out of town, it is likely cost-prohibitive to pay for the airfare for seminar helpers. Instead, include a notation in your flier that if people are interested in helping at the seminar, they may receive 50 percent tuition. Then, about 45 to 60 minutes prior to the seminar, train them in the needed duties (e.g., registration, CE certificates). Most seminars need only one or two helpers.

Printing Costs

One of the greatest expenses when conducting a seminar is the printing expense for brochures. It is very inexpensive to use a copy machine and make brochures in black and white. However, low quality brochures suggest a low quality seminar. A well-written, color brochure creates a positive first impression. If you plan on conducting only a few seminars, pay a printing company to make your brochures. Submit a request for bids to several printers and make a choice. If you find that you want to pursue the seminar business, consider purchasing a high-quality, color laser printer. The printing quality rivals professional printers if you develop your desktop publishing skills.

SEMINARS TO THE PUBLIC

There are seemingly limitless opportunities to conduct public seminars, whether your intent is to build up your practice through (a) future referrals or (b) provide a public service. The possibilities are only limited by your creativity, time, and motivation. Some seminars serve all of these purposes.

Future Referrals

Seminars intended to increase your client load are typically conducted in a location near your practice. We are clearly living in an age of convenience, and the costs of transportation have changed how far clients are willing to travel for ongoing appointments. A 1-hour appointment with a client for you, the therapist, involves much more than an hour's time for the client, who must travel to and from the appointment and may have other costs such as transportation (e.g., gas, bus, parking), the bother of asking others for a ride, babysitting, lost time at work, and in some cases much physical discomfort. A 1-hour appointment with you could easily amount to several hours of the client's time. Therefore, focus your advertising toward people who are most likely to make the necessary sacrifices to come to your practice. People who live several miles away might come to a seminar; however, their probability of returning on a weekly basis for therapy is much smaller.

The focus of your seminars should combine the client's needs with the services you offer. There is an advertising component. Be careful to spend more time discussing how clients' needs can be met, relative to the benefits offered by your clinic. If your presentation is informative, hits a chord emotionally and intellectually, and if the location of your business is convenient, you won't have to spend much time discussing the virtues of your practice. That is, focus on the clients, not you. Your warmness, personality, professionalism, and dedication will attract clients to your practice much more than a list of college degrees and profession associations.

Public Service

Seminars intended to provide a public service do not have an advertising component. They are intended to represent the profession as a whole, rather than attract clients to a specific clinic or practice. There are numerous potential locations to provide informational seminars as a public service. Opportunities include community centers, religious institutions, and special interest groups (e.g., cancer survivors; parents of children with ADHD, Multiple Sclerosis) typically have monthly meetings where a speaker is welcome.

Even though no direct advertising takes place, referrals are often generated after the seminar via audience questions about the speaker's availability. That is, speak to the audience about the benefits of your topic, not your clinic. If they are impressed with you and what you have to say, they will come. Providing simply your name and clinic affiliation is plenty of information for all of them to get in touch with you.

CONSULTING

Consulting referrals come from experience and reputation. Simply hanging a shingle that you consult to other professionals will not work. Consulting work usually comes through positive references, which in turn build your reputation. However, some mental health professionals advertise their consulting services to businesses, other professionals, and organizations.

I often provide consultation to other professionals in areas of documentation, clinic growth, and professional ethics. The source of referrals initially began after conducting a seminar. Often, after a seminar, a few people will contact you to consult on the topic. Overall, the more public speaking and writing you are involved in, the more your efforts will lead to consultations. I have never advertised as a consultant because word of mouth is perhaps the strongest advertising available.

There are no established fees for consulting, other than what the market will bear. I suggest your minimum consulting hourly fee be equal to your professional fee as a therapist. However, it is not uncommon to charge 1.5 to 2 times this fee for professional consulting.

TEACHING

Teaching college either part time or as an adjunct, in addition to running a practice, can be much more than simply an extra source of income. It provides numerous personal and professional rewards that cannot be found in any other endeavor. Some of the main benefits include keeping abreast in the field, opportunities for research, developing collegial relationships, a sense of helping others, professional opportunities, and as well as being personally rewarding. Although the pay is usually not much motivation, the other benefits are priceless.

Example of Wise Teaching Advice

I have taught at various colleges and universities since the early 1980s. Perhaps the greatest advice I ever received was from a nun, Sister Mary Aquinas Szott, at Felician College, a Catholic college in Lodi, New Jersey. When I was hired, she shared the following with me (paraphrased):

"When you teach a class, you are in the front of the room doing most of the talking and receiving most of the attention, but it is not about you. Don't ever let it be about you. It is about the students. They are here to learn. You are here for them; they are not here because of you. Give them all you have to offer, and don't expect anything from them. If you do this, the rewards are endless."

Lesson: Her advice places the professor in the role of a professional helper who is dedicated to students, not to personal gratification. Teaching is about giving, not receiving. It takes the professor off of the ivory tower to a place of professional humility and provides an excellent example of a role model.

There might be several therapists in your area who desire to teach, and some adjunct or part-time positions can be fairly competitive. The following points may help in securing a position amongst the competition

1. Apply for teaching positions (adjunct, part-time) at every college and university in your area, whether or not they are advertising for a position. Many adjunct positions are not advertised.

2. In an addendum to your cover letter and vita, list the courses you are able to teach. If it is your first time teaching, be sure to list general courses such as Introduction to Psychology, Counseling, Sociology, and so on. If you have a specialty, highlight your experience in the field. For example, if you specialize in Child Development, emphasize your interest in developmental and lifespan courses. Do not say that you can teach anything.

3. Contact the head of the department personally to discuss future teaching opportunities. Simply leaving a vita will assure your application is placed in a high pile of others. About 2 to 3 months before the beginning of the term, recontact the department head to discuss any possible openings.

4. Do your best to be available to teach during any hours. You may be required to adjust your professional schedule to accommodate teaching. If you are not able to make these adjustments, teaching might not be for you.

5. Offer to be a guest lecturer for a class that emphasizes your specialty. For example, a course in general psychology covers many topics, and you could be quite helpful for a class or two.

6. If you find that your lack of teaching experience hinders you from obtaining a position, gain experience in other areas of your field, such as at your state professional association or seminars (see previous section).

7. When you are offered an interview, be prepared. It is helpful to read a textbook about the topic area to ensure you are knowledgeable of current information. Never overstate your qualifications in an interview. Your expertise is certainly important, but emphasize your interest in teaching, not your expertise. Your expertise will speak for itself. However, do not put yourself down, as you may appear to have low self-esteem.

8. Typically, a first teaching position can be easier to land at smaller schools, such as community colleges and small private colleges.

9. Once you are hired, be sure to clearly follow the school's policies, procedures, and deadlines. Be an expert in what you know about the field, but also be humble about being the new person on the block. Follow the examples of other faculty in areas such as a course syllabi, attendance policies, grading procedures, level of course difficulty, and availability to students. Experienced faculty do not appreciate "know it alls."

10. Always be emotionally supportive to students, but keep a professional distance. Students, individually and in groups, will test your boundaries.

11. Your chances of being rehired will depend on how well you fit into the system, informal faculty opinions, student evaluations, and a lack of complaints. Therefore, give it your all.

12. Faculty who receive the highest student ratings tend to be personable, interesting, available, knowledgeable, fair, and open-minded. They provide interesting real-world examples and use a variety of teaching methods. It is all about giving of yourself and what you know.

PROFESSIONAL ASSOCIATIONS

All states have professional associations for mental health professionals. Each association has an organizational structure in which administrative personnel are composed of association members. Some positions, such as the president, are elected, while others are voluntary. Slowly working your way up in a professional association gives you valuable administrative experience, leadership opportunities, and a sense of camaraderie. In addition, it may provide stepping stones for future leadership within the organization as well as consulting opportunities as your reputation increases.

VOLUNTEERING

Volunteer opportunities exist in some form wherever there are people in need. Your amount of involvement may range from occasionally helping out to being placed on a schedule. Ongoing services may be conducted in places such as nursing homes, shelters, halfway houses, crisis shelters, or free clinics. The experience is rewarding and may lead to future, formal referrals. Emergency counseling volunteer opportunities, along with valuable crisis training, can be found at the Red Cross and may lead to valuable networking.

SUMMARY

A professional reputation starts with humility and the demeanor of a student. Those who are the most accomplished in the field are typically listeners rather than talkers and do not seek recognition. Hard work, ethics, consistency, innovation, keeping up professionally, and trying to be part of a team are the key ingredients to developing a good professional reputation.

One who seeks recognition and a reputation as an accomplished professional will likely not get very far in the field. Self-promotion is unappealing to others. People do not like following a self-centered leader.

When you begin your career, view it as the beginning of your education. Do not present yourself as an accomplished professional. Very little of what you practice in mental health is learned in graduate school. Therefore, seek as much supervision and guidance as possible from an experienced, accomplished mentor. Help out in professional activities such as seminars, presentations, and staff trainings, but do not present yourself as higher than your level of experience. Give yourself at least a few years of learning before presenting yourself as an expert.

TEST YOUR KNOWLEDGE

1. Which of the following behaviors could end a therapist's career?

    (a) Billing errors

    (b) Charging the maximum fee

    (c) Using a collection agency

    (d) Double billing

2. Which of the following is seemingly minor, but could lead to a decreased reputation if repeated enough?

    (a) Sexual contact with a client

    (b) Tardiness for appointments

    (c) Collecting co-payments

    (d) Adhering to policies and procedures

3. Therapists desiring to set up their own seminar should be

    (a) professionally qualified.

    (b) confident in their speaking skills.

(c) able to negotiate.

(d) all of these.

4. This text suggests that if you apply for an initial teaching position you emphasize your

(a) coursework.

(b) professional experience.

(c) desire to teach.

(d) publications.

Answers: 1. d; 2. b; 3. d; 4. c

7

Effective Time Management

YOUR TIME—SETTING PRIORITIES

Many mental health professionals are reluctant to talk about money. They are the first to say that money is not their priority because they are in the field to help clients. However, if little or no thought is given to finances, a practice will not stay in business, and no more clients will be helped. Clearly, time is money. Effective time management requires strict personal discipline and strong managerial skills. Without managing time wisely, many necessary tasks important for clinic growth will be procrastinated.

Whatever the size of the clinic, a specific amount of time must be devoted to a number of priority areas. These include time with clients, supervision, administrative tasks, public relations, and advertising. If too much time is devoted to seeing clients, there might not be enough time devoted to increasing new business. If too much time is spent on administrative activities, there might not be enough current clients to keep up financially. Clearly, a balance of clinical responsibilities is needed to maintain the present and future stability of the clinic.

Clinic directors or managers do much more than make clinical and financial decisions. Budgeting is not simply making financial decisions, but also involving leadership in the clinic's budgeting of time. This skill involves much more than scheduling. It also involves motivating therapists to devote a portion of their time to clinic enhancing activities that do not necessarily produce direct income. The most successful clinics function as a unit or a team, in which effective leadership is the key.

TIMING OF THERAPY SESSIONS

Simply devoting time to internal clinic activities is not enough. Time management is also very important in ongoing therapy sessions. A simple decision to schedule clients every 45 minutes, instead of every 60 minutes, can be beneficial to everyone involved. For example, if two therapists decide to see clients from 9:00 A.M. until 12:00 P.M., it is possible that one therapist would see three clients, while the other therapist would see four clients in the same time period.

By seeing extra clients in this 3-hour period, one is able to either produce more income or see fewer clients on other days in order to devote more time to other responsibilities. I do not suggest scheduling clients all day, 45 minutes apart, for back-to-back sessions. This could lead to overloading oneself. But if 1 hour or more per day can be saved, the time is well managed. If only one more client is seen per day, 5 days per week for 50 weeks, there is a potential of 250 additional client hours per year, resulting in additional billing of $25,000 yearly if the fee is $100 per hour. A small practice with five therapists using this method (one extra client per day, without an additional total time) would bill an additional $125,000 per year for the practice. Two extra clients per day would double this amount. Changing a clinical session (or clinical hour) from 60 to 45 minutes and charging for an hour is not fraudulent. A clinical hour is defined as 45–50 minutes, not 60 minutes. Forty-five minutes is typically plenty of time to conduct a session of therapy. The key is to stay on target and stick with the treatment plan and the client's needs. It may be helpful to inform the client when there are

	Client 1	Client 2	Client 3	Client 4	Lunch
Therapist 1	9:00–10:00	10:00–11:00	11:00–12:00	None	12:00–X
Therapist 2	9:00–9:45	9:45–10:30	10:30–11:15	11:15–12:00	12:00–X

Transitioning from a 60- to a 45-Minute Session

Provide training in how to keep on track during a session. Practice and teach skills for staying focused by role-playing various scenarios in which the client does not focus, or wants to change the topic to chit-chat or unhelpful material. Work on staying within the treatment plan and keeping the session therapeutic. Plenty of material can be covered in 45 minutes. Typically, therapists who state that they must use a full 60 minutes are able to gradually adjust to a 45-minute session after both they and their clients have accommodated to the change. However, do not become upset if some therapists insist on providing 60-minute sessions. Some schools of thought and personalities require more time per session than others.

Example of the Effects of Running Late in Sessions

I once worked with a therapist who scheduled clients on the hour. He regularly overran sessions by about 20 or more minutes. If every client showed up, by the end of the day, the therapist was typically over 1 hour late for the last appointment and did not have time for a lunch hour or any breaks. Often, clients in the waiting room became quite upset and sometimes left and never returned to the clinic. Good time management is part of customer service.

5 minutes left in the session. Then there is no need to end the session abruptly at 45 minutes.

Too many people work hard but not smart. That is, they work long hours, but too much time is wasted on activities that benefit neither their clients nor themselves. The more productive and time efficient you are at work, the more time you will have for nonwork activities.

NINE PRACTICAL WAYS TO SAVE TIME

Write Progress Notes during the Session

Many therapists conduct a session of psychotherapy in 45 minutes, and spend the next 15 minutes writing progress notes. There is nothing wrong with this procedure, but that 15 minutes could have been spent either with another client, fulfilling other clinic responsibilities, or relaxing.

Although it might take a little getting used to, writing progress notes during the session has many benefits beyond saving time. When progress notes are written during the session, the therapist does not have to rely on trying to remember specifically what transpired during the session. It is very difficult to remember nonverbal clinical observations, client quotes, or other important details unless they are written as they happen.

Progress notes do not have to be a literary work of art. They are simply remarks on client behavior, clinical observations, and treatment strategies that provide evidence of what took place in the session. They help validate the diagnosis and ongoing impairments and the progress of respective treatment. See Chapter 10.

The process of writing progress notes during the session can indirectly tell clients that what they say is important. It takes up no session time because they are being written as the client speaks. Typically, the bulk of progress notes is simple sentences and phrases, so the therapist does not lose focus on what the client is saying. When the client leaves the session, the documentation is complete. The therapist does not have to spend time at the end of the session, or at the end of the day or week, catching up on progress notes. The therapist is ready to see another client immediately after the session or take a break before seeing the next client.

Do Not Schedule Long Lunch Breaks

Yes, therapists should eat and have time to relax. However, it is the experience of most therapists that about 15 to 25 percent of their appointments are no-shows or cancellations. Perhaps the highest rate of no-show clients are intakes. If you work in a typical practice that has a fair amount of no-shows, consider having lunch or taking breaks when there are no-shows. If you regularly schedule your lunch, for example, at the noon hour, it is quite possible that you could have seen a client then and eaten your lunch at another time.

Although this practice may be inconvenient, it can potentially add another client to your load every day. If eating out with other people at a set time is very important to you, go ahead and take a scheduled lunch hour, or consider a scheduled lunch about half the time, rather than daily. If you work in a setting without no-shows, go ahead and schedule your lunch break.

If at All Possible, Start Early in the Morning

For some reason, many therapists are late risers. Few clinics have early morning hours. Many parents who work all day do not want to give up evening or workday time to come to therapy. People will often come to an early morning appointment such as 7:00 or 8:00 A.M. Some therapists quickly tire of working evening hours when they become accustomed to getting out early due to working morning hours.

Some clients prefer early morning hours. They tend to be a little more obsessive about not missing work, so they come in beforehand. And some parents will take their children to counseling early in the morning so they don't miss school in the middle of the day and don't have to give up evening time.

Do Not Write Treatment Plans Outside of the Session

Treatment plans are intended to be written via an active process between the therapist and the client. The goals and objectives are to be written collaboratively with the client. Some third-party payers and accrediting agencies want written evidence that the treatment plan was conducted in this manner. You are wasting time that could be very helpful to the client unless you write the treatment plan together during the second session.

A well-written treatment plan can be very therapeutic in that it enables the client to learn and understand what will take place in therapy and what progress can be expected in a given period of time. If you have three new intakes per week, you will save 3 hours time by formulating and writing the treatment plan during the session.

All documentation that pertains to therapy (assessment, treatment plans, and progress notes) should be written during the session, with the client's participation (within the parameters of the situation). However, do not perform administrative tasks within the session because they are not therapeutic and would constitute fraudulent billing. Documentation, with the clients corroboration, can be quite therapeutic and provides immediate, helpful feedback to the client.

Learn Your Billing Codes Well

Chapter 8 provides a primer for billing. Without a thorough knowledge of billing codes, it is very easy to make errors. If a therapist is not aware of billing codes that are assigned to tasks such as the explanation of findings, interpreting tests, providing feedback, receiving information when the client is not present, or other factors mentioned in Chapter 8, it is quite possible to bill under a wrong code and not be paid or mistakenly decide that a service is not billable when it actually could be paid.

Learn How to Dictate Your Reports

If part of your job is to produce typed reports, treatment plans, or any other documentation, it is likely not worth your time to type them yourself. Typically, therapists charge over $100 per hour, while typists charge a significantly lower amount. A person well experienced in dictating a report can usually dictate about one page per minute. It will take a typist about 4 to 5 minutes to accurately type one page. Dictation services are not expensive. Some larger clinics have clerical staff who service this function. The time a therapist can save by having someone else type their reports can easily lead to saving enough time to see a few more clients per week. Using a dictation service is very cost-effective when the time saved is well

Example of a Therapist with Billing Problems

I recently spent several weeks supervising a fellow psychologist who was told by an insurance company that he overbilled. He sought training in the documentation of billing procedures and billing codes.

His concerns stemmed from an intake and testing he conducted for a minor. He sent the minor into a room to take a test and interviewed the parent at the same time. When the client's parent received the report of services from the insurance company, it notes that 5 hours of services were being charged. The parent phoned the insurance company, complaining that they were at the office for no more than 3 hours, not 5.

The problem was the therapist used the billing code 90801 for the entire 5 hours, which is designated as the therapist providing direct testing services. He called the 5 hours an intake. The actual timing and billing codes are as follows:

Code 90801	Diagnostic Interview	1.0 hrs
96101	IQ test (therapist with client)	1.0 hrs
90846	Collaboration with parents	1.0 hrs
96101	Client filled out Minnesota Multiphasic Personality Inventory–Adolescent (separate room)	1.0 hrs
90889 or 96101	Interpretation of tests (outside of session)	1.0 hrs
Total time spent (client and parent)		5.0 hrs
Actual time client and parent were at the office		3.0 hrs
Overlap of time (client and father, separate rooms)		1.0 hrs

utilized. Confidentiality is preserved by having the transcriptionist sign a confidentiality agreement.

Use a Billing Service if There Is No Staff on Hand to Bill for You

The same logic applies as mentioned for learning to dictate your reports. That is, the amount that you pay for a billing service is much

---

Example of Time and Money Saved by Having Others Type Your Reports

I conduct several psychological evaluations each week. I have found that when I type one of my reports, it takes at least 45 minutes. However, when I dictate the same report, it takes no more 10 minutes. Translated into the cost benefits for 10 reports, the following is noted:

	Cost	Additional Income
10 reports by dictation services	$200	
Time of 45 min × 10 reports is 450 min – 100 min of dictation time. The net saved time is 350 min, which translates to about 7.5, 45 min sessions. 7.5 × $100 = $750.		$750
Net additional gain after about 7.5 client visits	($750–200) = $550	

---

less than the amount you could be making by using that time conducting professional services or expanding your business.

When Holding Staff Meetings, Have a Clear, Time-Limited Agenda

Prepare an outline and supply any handout materials needed to organize the meeting efficiently. If there is little to discuss in an upcoming meeting, cancel it and work on clinic enriching activities. Do not hold staff meetings simply because they are scheduled. Other staff will appreciate knowing that meetings take place only when necessary.

Practice Effective Time Management of Office Space

A common concern in many growing clinics is distribution of office space. If each therapist has a separate office, there is no problem with time conflicts, but when a clinic grows, it cannot obtain a new office each time a therapist is hired. If the average, full-time thera-

> *Example of Effective Office-Space Time Management*
>
> I managed a clinic where there were 25 offices and almost 50 therapists. With a monthly lease amount of several thousand dollars, adding more offices was not possible.
>
> Senior therapists were given their choice of offices, but were required to state their working times. During times they were not seeing clients, new and part-time therapists were available to schedule clients. The net result was an increase in the potential office-space time available by about 50 percent, leading to a significant increase in the number of clients seen.
>
> Some of the senior therapists were upset that someone was using their office, but most clinicians realized that the move was in the best interest of the clients and clinic.

pist sees 20 to 25 clients per week and the clinic is open about 40 to 66 hours per week, there is much wasted office space. It is better to manage office hours than to allow only one therapist per office.

SUMMARY

Therapists must balance their time between clinical and administrative duties. Balancing the clinical and administrative duties leads to both maintaining an adequate client load, obtaining new business, and keeping up with required documentation requirements.

When therapists place too much time attending either clinical or administrative duties, the other will suffer. For example, if a therapist spends too much time with clients and does not take care of other responsibilities such as administrative tasks, documentation, public relations, and clinic-building activities, there will be no additional clients.

There are procedures that can free up time for the therapist to either see more clients or devote to other duties. Time saving procedures such as writing progress notes and the treatment plan during the session, and ending sessions at a 45-minute clinical hour, result in having more time available for providing additional services or other duties.

Habits such as waiting until after a session to take care of basic paperwork tasks or extending the length of sessions leads to getting behind in paperwork, decreased administrative and clinic-building activities, and having less available personal time.

Learning billing codes well and following ethical billing procedures will prevent billing and ethical concerns. Following ethical billing procedures, and being aware of which billing codes are allowed by the various third-party payers also helps build up a positive reputation and increases referrals.

Problematic or excessive billing to third parties may lead to lost contracts. Excessive billing can also lead to client complaints and ethical issues.

TEST YOUR KNOWLEDGE

1. True or False? It is possible to legally and ethically see four clients for 4 clinical hours of billing in 3 clock hours.

    (a) True

    (b) False

2. This book suggests that therapists in an outpatient mental health clinic consider not scheduling a specific time for a lunch break because

    (a) therapists need to work all day long.

    (b) typically there are a number of no-show appointments or cancellations, and a break can be taken during that time.

3. This book suggests that therapists who need reports typed do which of the following?

    (a) Hire the cheapest transcriptionist available.

    (b) Never hire a transcriptionist. It is a breach of confidentiality.

    (c) Never hire a transcriptionist. Type reports in your off time.

    (d) Hire a transcriptionist, and perform clinical or administrative duties in the time saved.

4. Why should a therapist learn billing codes?

    (a) Therapists do not need to learn billing codes. The biller does that.

    (b) There are many combinations of procedures and people in a session, and only the therapist knows for sure how session time was used.

    (c) Therapists, even in large clinics, do their own billing.

    (d) They are ultimately responsible for what is billed.

    (e) Two of these.

5. What is the main advantage of writing progress notes and treatment plans during the session?

    (a) There is no advantage. It takes away from session time.

    (b) The information is more accurate because it is here and now.

    (c) It increases the time with the client.

    (d) It allows you to attend to the client more.

Answers: 1. a; 2. b; 3. d; 4. e; 5. b

Part B

Administrative and Documentation Procedures

8

Billing Procedures

Any successful business must have clear and specific policies and procedures regarding the collection of funds. Policies are written guidelines, while procedures are steps and guidelines to follow the policies. Mental health professionals are rarely trained in business principles and often neglect pursuing debt collection. New therapists may assume that clients will pay their bill or, if a client produces an insurance card, that payment is assured. This is clearly not the case. Whether the responsible payer is the client or a third-party, payment is never a surety.

To complicate matters, different insurance companies have different policies and procedures for payment. Without awareness of their provisions, it can be difficult to collect the amounts billed to them. When the client's insurance company denies payment, there are means of rebilling, but when no payment is received the clinic must either bill the client or excuse the bill.

Too many excused bills can lead to several problems, such as therapists not being paid if they are paid on commission and not meeting the clinic's financial obligations. This results in a high turnover of therapists, poor morale, and financial concerns.

Many, if not most, therapists seem to have difficulty asking clients for money. They prefer to deal with their clients' emotional and psychological needs and view themselves as helpers. When financial concerns come up, they believe those issues may lead to ill feelings that could harm the relationship and result in the client not returning for services. Thus, the bills pile up. This can easily be prevented when a clinic abides by a financial policy.

Some therapists are assertive enough to be sure that their clients pay for services each session. They emphasize the importance of being responsible and treat payments in a manner similar to an MD's office, where there is typically a strictness about collecting fees. In my experience, most therapists who are reticent to collect money from clients become disillusioned about the field when their income depends on fees received, but their accounts receivable are quite high. It is very important that clinic management provides ample training to therapists in collecting fees. Larger clinics often do not require therapists to collect fees because they have people assigned to this task. Clients must first check in and take care of financial matters, prior to seeing the therapist.

PAYMENT CONTRACTS WITH CLIENTS

Payment contracts with clients are necessary for a clinic's financial survival. The contract specifically spells out the responsible party, fees, and policies and procedures for collecting unpaid funds. Forms such as payment contracts must be filled out before services begin. Typically, clients are asked to come in to fill out forms about 30 to 60 minutes prior to their initial session.

A written copy of the clinic's financial policy, along with a payment contract for services, should be signed by each client. It is suggested that the clinic's financial policy clearly covers the following information:

1. Designation of the person responsible for payment. This is especially important when there are issues of custody and support. Typically, the parent who transports or accompanies the child to the clinic is the person responsible for payment, unless the other parent signs the payment contract.

2. A notation that the insurance company is not ultimately responsible for payment; thus, if the insurance company does not pay, or does not pay in a timely manner, the person responsible for payment will be billed.

3. A description of how insurance or third-party payers are billed.

4. Time limits as to how long the clinic will wait for third-party payments before the client is financially responsible.

5. Interest rates charged for late payments.

6. Collection of insurance co-payments and deductibles.

7. Assignment of insurance benefits.

8. Policies regarding missed appointments.

9. Policies for receiving services when the client's unpaid balance reaches a given level.

10. Policies regarding payment when children come to the interview without a payment or prearranged financial agreement.

11. A signature from the person responsible for payment.

A payment contract is a legal document and should be reviewed by an attorney prior to use. It should be written within the guidelines of the Federal Truth in Lending Act, including specific information such as the cost of specific services, late fees, and interest rates. Although somewhat redundant with your financial policy, specifically cover costs such as no-show fees, and ensure a clear designation of the person responsible for payment of services (who must sign the contract). Refer to the financial policy in the form. Be sure that both forms are signed. Without this contract, it can be very difficult to collect delinquent fees. At a minimum, it should contain the following provisions:

1. Client's full name and demographic information.

2. The name and demographics of the person responsible for payment. Many collection agencies request that you also receive this person's social security number, plus the name and address of their employer. This information helps significantly when use of a collection agency is necessary.

3. Payment rates (hourly fees) for each service intended to be conducted (e.g., testing, initial evaluation, counseling [individual, group, family, etc.]).

4. Insurance deductible amount.

5. Insurance co-payment amounts.

6. Policy limits.

7. A disclaimer that the client, not the clinic, is responsible for fees not collected by third parties.

8. References to the financial policy.

BILLING INSURANCE COMPANIES

Most insurance companies require a 1500 form. Some allow for online billing, while others receive the form by fax or mail. Several customizable billing programs are available that coordinate with the 1500 form.

WHAT TO DO WHEN PAYMENT IS REJECTED

Therapists are often surprised by the number of insurance claims that are initially rejected. Even the most seemingly minor error or deletion may result in a rejection. However, a rejection for payment does not mean that you can't get paid. There are multiple reasons, most of which are clerical, that an insurance company denies payment.

When a rejection is received, it is accompanied by a rejection code. The code sometimes is self-explanatory, and the error can usually be amended by noting the reason for the rejection and making appropriate corrections. Typical mistakes are incorrect Current Procedural Terminology (CPT) codes, incorrect spelling of a name, incorrect insurance numbers, or any number of typos.

If you plan on doing your own billing, you must stay attuned to billing code changes. For example, the 96100 code for testing was replaced by 3 codes, 96101, 96102, and 96103, to more easily clarify who conducted the testing. However, even after several months, therapists keep using the 96100 billing code and keep receiving rejection notices.

When you are unsure of why a bill was rejected, phone the third-party payer. They can look up the claim and explain why it was rejected. Oftentimes, during your discussion, they will discover that the claim should have been paid. In such cases it will still have to be rebilled.

BILLING CODES

CPT-4 Codes

Not all insurance companies cover all billing codes.

Code No.	Brief Description
90801	Psychiatric diagnostic interview examination
90802	Interactive psychiatric interview using play equipment, physical devices, language interpreter, or other mechanisms of communication
90804	Individual psychotherapy; insight-oriented, behavior modifying and/or supportive, in an office or outpatient facility, approximately 20 to 30 minutes face-to-face with patient
90805	Individual psychotherapy; insight-oriented, behavior modifying and/or supportive, in an office or outpatient facility with medical evaluation and management services, approximately 20 to 30 minutes face-to-face with patient
90806	Individual psychotherapy; insight-oriented, behavior modifying and/or supportive, in an office or outpatient facility, approximately 45 to 50 minutes face-to-face with patient
90807	Individual psychotherapy; insight-oriented, behavior modifying and/or supportive, in an office or outpatient facility with medical evaluation and management services, approxi-

mately 45 to 50 minutes face-to-face with patient

90810   Individual psychotherapy, interactive, using play equipment, physical devices, language interpreter, or other mechanisms of nonverbal communication, in an office or outpatient facility, approximately 75 to 80 minutes face-to-face with patient

90811   Individual psychotherapy, interactive, using play equipment, physical devices, language interpreter, or other mechanisms of nonverbal communication, in an office or outpatient facility, with medical evaluation and management services, approximately 75 to 80 minutes face-to-face with patient

90812   Individual psychotherapy, interactive, using play equipment, physical devices, language interpreter, or other mechanisms of nonverbal communication, in an office or outpatient facility, approximately 45 to 50 minutes face-to-face with patient

90813   Individual psychotherapy, interactive, using play equipment, physical devices, language interpreter, or other mechanisms of nonverbal communication, in an office or outpatient facility, with medical evaluation and management services, approximately 45 to 50 minutes face-to-face with patient

90814   Individual psychotherapy, interactive, using play equipment, physical devices, language interpreter, or other mechanisms of nonverbal communication, in an office or outpatient facility, approximately 75 to 80 minutes face-to-face with patient

90815   Individual psychotherapy, interactive, using play equipment, physical devices, language interpreter, or other mechanisms of nonverbal communication, in an office or outpatient facility, with medical evaluation and management services, approximately 75 to 80 minutes face-to-face with patient

90816   Individual psychotherapy, insight oriented, behavior modifying and/or supportive, in an inpatient hospital, partial hospital, or residential care setting, approximately 20 to 30 minutes face-to-face with the patient

90817   Individual psychotherapy, insight oriented, behavior modifying and/or supportive, in an inpatient hospital, partial hospital, or residential care setting with medical evaluation and management services, approximately 20 to 30 minutes face-to-face with the patient

90818   Individual psychotherapy, insight oriented, behavior modifying and/or supportive, in an inpatient hospital, partial hospital, or residential care setting, approximately 45 to 50 minutes face-to-face with the patient

90820   Individual psychotherapy, insight oriented, behavior modifying and/or supportive, in an inpatient hospital, partial hospital, or residential care setting with medical evaluation and management services, approximately 45 to 50 minutes face-to-face with the patient

90821   Individual psychotherapy, insight oriented, behavior modifying and/or supportive, in an inpatient hospital, partial hospital, or residential care setting, approximately 75 to 80 minutes face-to-face with the patient

90822   Individual psychotherapy, insight oriented, behavior modifying and/or supportive, in an inpatient hospital, partial hospital, or residential care setting with medical evaluation

	and management services, approximately 75 to 80 minutes face-to-face with the patient
90823	Individual psychotherapy, interactive, using play equipment, physical devices, language interpreter, or other mechanisms of nonverbal communication, in an inpatient hospital or residential care setting, approximately 20 to 30 minutes face-to-face with the patient
90824	Individual psychotherapy, interactive, using play equipment, physical devices, language interpreter, or other mechanisms of nonverbal communication, in an inpatient hospital or residential care setting, with medical evaluation and management services, approximately 20 to 30 minutes face-to-face with the patient
90826	Individual psychotherapy, interactive, using play equipment, physical devices, language interpreter, or other mechanisms of nonverbal communication, in an inpatient hospital or residential care setting, approximately 45 to 50 minutes face-to-face with the patient
90827	Individual psychotherapy, interactive, using play equipment, physical devices, language interpreter, or other mechanisms of nonverbal communication, in an inpatient hospital or residential care setting, with medical evaluation and management services, approximately 45 to 50 minutes face-to-face with the patient
90828	Individual psychotherapy, interactive, using play equipment, physical devices, language interpreter, or other mechanisms of nonverbal communication, in an inpatient hospital or residential care setting, approximately 75 to 80 minutes face-to-face with the patient

90829	Individual psychotherapy, interactive, using play equipment, physical devices, language interpreter, or other mechanisms of nonverbal communication, in an inpatient hospital or residential care setting, with medical evaluation and management services, approximately 75 to 80 minutes face-to-face with the patient
90845	Psychoanalysis
90846	Family psychotherapy (without the patient present)
90847	Family psychotherapy (conjoint psychotherapy, with patient present)
90849	Multiple-family group psychotherapy
90853	Group psychotherapy (other than a multiple-family group)
90857	Interactive group psychotherapy
90862	Pharmacologic management, including prescription, use, and review of medication with no more than minimal medical psychotherapy
90865	Narcosynthesis for psychiatric diagnostic and therapeutic purposes (e.g., sodium amobarbital [amytal] review)
90870	Electroconvulsive therapy (includes necessary monitoring); single seizure
90871	Electroconvulsive therapy (includes necessary monitoring); multiple seizures per day
90875	Individual psychophysiological therapy incorporating biofeedback training by any modality (face-to-face with the patient), with psychotherapy (e.g., insight-oriented, behavior modifying, or supportive psychotherapy); approximately 20 to 30 minutes

90876	Individual psychophysiological therapy incorporating biofeedback training by any modality (face-to-face with the patient), with psychotherapy (e.g., insight-oriented, behavior modifying, or supportive psychotherapy); approximately 45 to 50 minutes
90880	Hypnotherapy
90882	Environmental intervention for medical management purposes on a psychiatric patient's behalf with agencies, employers, or institutions
90885	Psychiatric evaluation of hospital records, other psychiatric reports, psychometric and/or projective tests, and other accumulated data for medical diagnostic purposes
90887	Interpretation or explanation of results of psychiatric, other medical examinations and procedures, or other accumulated data to family for other persons, or advising them how to assist patient
90889	Preparation of report of patient's psychiatric status, history, treatment, or progress (other than for legal consultative purposes) for other physicians, agencies, or insurance carriers
90899	Unlisted psychiatric service or procedure

Psychologists now have a more accurate, refined way of billing for services provided to patients with a physical health diagnosis, thanks to the advent of six new reimbursement codes under the CPT coding system. As of January 1, 2002, codes for health and behavior assessment and intervention services now apply to behavioral, social, and psychophysiological procedures for the prevention, treatment, or management of physical health problems. Until now, almost all intervention codes used by psychologists involved psychotherapy and required a mental health diagnosis, such as under the *DSM-IV.* In contrast, health and behavior assessment and intervention services focus on patients whose primary diagnosis is physical in nature. Use of the codes will enable reimbursement for the delivery of psychological services for an individual whose problem is a physical illness and who does not have a mental health diagnosis.

96150	The initial assessment of the patient to determine the biological, psychological, and social factors affecting the patient's physical health and any treatment problems.
96151	Reassessment of the patient to evaluate the patient's condition and determine the need for further treatment. A reassessment may be performed by a clinician other than the one who conducted the patient's initial assessment.
96152	The intervention service provided to an individual to modify the psychological, behavioral, cognitive, and social factors affecting the patient's physical health and well-being. Examples include increasing the patient's awareness about his or her disease and using cognitive and behavioral approaches to initiate physician prescribed diet and exercise regimens.
96153	The intervention service provided to a group. An example is a smoking cessation program that includes educational information, cognitive-behavioral treatment, and social support. Group sessions typically last for 90 minutes and involve 8 to 10 patients.
96154	The intervention service provided to a family with the patient present. For example, a psychologist could use relaxation techniques with both a diabetic child and his or her parents to reduce the child's fear of receiving injections and the parents' tension when administering the injections.

96155   The intervention service provided to a family without the patient present. An example would be working with parents and siblings to shape the diabetic child's behavior, such as praising successful diabetes management behaviors and ignoring disruptive tactics.

The typical minimum client information to supply a billing service is as follows:

Client's full name, address, phone

Client's Social Security number

Policyholder's full name

Date of birth

Date(s) of services

Insurance policy number (including group number)

Numerical code for each diagnosis on the appropriate axis

Numerical code for the type(s) of services for each date of service

The time spent for each services (typically in 1 hour units, but may vary)

Authorization or preapproval numbers

Names and policy numbers of other insurances

BILLING PRIMER

Whether the client is an insurance client or a cash client, certain administrative intake information, which goes beyond the necessary required information for billers, should be collected. The worst-case scenario is that the client's insurance company preapproves services. Then after several sessions are conducted, no payment comes in, payment is ultimately rejected, and the client refuses to pay. Unfortunately, this scenario is not uncommon. When insurance or managed care companies authorize services, they typically include a disclaimer that payment is not guaranteed. Their initial authorization is based on information known at the time of the authorization, but it is subject to change.

As a clinic director or manager, there must be policies in place that protect the clinic from nonpayment of funds. The simple solution is to readily inform the client that you provide insurance billing as a service, but if the client's insurance does not pay, the client is responsible for payment.

No clinic desires to take a client to collections. It clearly destroys

---

Example of the Benefits of Having a Clear Collection Policy

A client requested counseling services. The clinic took insurance information over the phone and verified benefits with the insurance company. After about six sessions, insurance rejection letters were received. The client stated that it must be an error. A phone call to the insurance company resulted in a request for more information. By the eighth session, another rejection letter was received. The client was upset and asked the clinic to appeal the decision to the insurance company. The appeal resulted in an affirmation of the rejection. The client then discontinued services.

Several bills were sent to the client, who never responded to any correspondence. After 90 days, the bill of over $1,000 was turned over to a collection agency. The client refused to pay the collection agency. The collection agency turned his name and the amount owed to the credit bureau, thus lowering his credit rating. A few months later, the client applied for a loan and was turned down. He checked his credit report and saw the nonpayment history. Immediately, the client phoned the clinic stating that he was going to sue the clinic because of a violation of confidentiality. He reasoned that the clinic gave his name to the collection agency and credit bureau, thus informing them that he received mental health services. He stressed that a clinic cannot reveal the name of its clients, thus the clinic was in trouble. He then offered to drop the suit if the bill was cancelled.

The clinic director then asked the ex-client to look over his signed payment contract, in which there were clauses that covered payment responsibilities when insurance does not pay, interest rates, the use of collection services, and what information would be given to the collection agencies who may turn in the information to the credit bureau. This information did not disclose any clinical information, only financial information. The client stated that he never signed such a contract and became more furious. The clinic then sent him a copy of the payment contract that stated each of these policies and verified that he understood them. Within a week he paid the bill.

the relationship with the client, but the clinic must stay in business. Financial policies for collections must be clearly communicated to the client before services begin. Clients should not be surprised that they are responsible when a third party does not pay. Financial policies must not be the fine print. There will be cases when you will decide not to pursue collections due to factors such as financial hardship or uncollectability of funds.

Other businesses do not quickly forgive clients who receive a valuable service and then refuse to pay. If we teach clients to be irresponsible financially, we are depriving them of being responsible for their actions. This is not good therapy!

Insurance Forms and Descriptions

The CMS-1500 claim form is the standard insurance claim form for most national insurance companies. The form comprises 33 blocks of information as follows:

Block #	Information Covered
1–13	Client and policy information
14–23	Diagnostic information, authorizations
24	Services dates, procedures, services, supplies
25–33	Provider information, charges for services

The following provides brief descriptions of what information is placed in the 33 blocks of the CMS-1500 form. Some insurance companies vary some of the procedures.

Blocks 1–13	Client and Policy Information
1	Check the type of insurance. If the insurer is any other, such as a national insurance company, check "other."
1A	Enter the insurance identification number. Do not place dashes. Spaces are okay if they appear on the insurance ID card.

2 Enter the insured person's name (first, last, middle) *exactly* how it appears on the ID card. If the person states that his or her name has recently changed, do not write the new name unless the change has been registered with the insurance company. First, validate that the change has previously been made with the insurance company.

3 Enter the clients date of birth in the MM/DD/YYYY (or YY) format, depending on the payee. Be sure to leave at least one space between the month, date, and year. Check the box indicating the patient's sex.

4 If the client and the policyholder are the same person, write *same*. If they are different people, fill in the policyholder's name (last, first, middle) exactly the same as noted on the insurance card or in the policy.

5 Lines 1 and 2. Enter the client's mailing address.
Line 3. Enter the client's five-digit zip code, area code, and phone number. Do not use parentheses or dashes.

6 Check the appropriate box indicating the client's relationship with the insured.

7 If the client and the policyholder are the same person, write *same*. If they are different people, fill in the policyholder's address.

8 Check the appropriate box that indicates the client's marital, employment, and student status. If the patient is a full-time student between the ages of 19 and 23, benefits will likely not be paid unless the insurance company is provided with proof from the school (usually from the registrar) of the student's full-time status each school term (semester,

trimester, quarter) of the school year in which insurance services are used. The student must be of full-time status at the time services were received.

9   This block is only used when the client has secondary insurance.
If there is secondary insurance, enter the name of the policyholder for the secondary insurance. If the person is the patient, enter *same*.

9A   Blank. If there is secondary insurance, enter the ID and group number of the secondary insurance.

9B   Blank. If there is secondary insurance, enter the secondary policyholder's date of birth in the MM/DD/YYYY (or YY) format. Be sure to leave at least one space between the month, date, and year. Check the box indicating the secondary policyholder's sex.

9C   Blank. If there is secondary insurance, enter the secondary policyholder's employer or school if the policy is an employee group health plan.

9D   Blank. If there is secondary insurance, enter the name of the secondary insurance plan.

10A–C   Mark an *X* to indicate whether the client's condition is due to employment, auto accident, or other accident.

10D   Blank. Various payers may use this line for specific reasons. Refer to their instructions.

11   Enter the policy group number if available.

11A   Enter the policyholder's date of birth in the MM/DD/YYYY (or YY) format. Be sure to leave at least one space between the month, date, and year. Check the box indicating the policyholder's sex.

11B	If the policy is an employer group health plan, enter the name of the employer as designated on the insurance card.
11C	Enter the insurance or program plan name.
11D	Enter *no* if there is not a secondary insurance. If there is secondary insurance enter *yes*.
12	Enter *signature on file* if the client has signed a release of information (that is on file) to the insurance company. If this release is not on file, the client must sign and date in the space provided.
13	Enter *signature on file* to indicate that the files contain the client's signature that payments will be sent to the provider. If the signature is not on file, the client must sign and date in the space provided for payments to be sent to the provider.

Blocks 14–23   Diagnostic Information, Authorizations

14	This block is typically used in medical situations for the onset date of the injury, illness, or pregnancy.
15	This block is used to enter the date of a prior episode of the same illness if this information is available.
16	If there is a known date when the client was not able to work, enter the date.
17	Enter the name and credentials of the referral physician or source of referral, if applicable.
17A	Enter the PIN number of the participating provider in line 17. If the source is a nonparticipating provider, enter the person's Social Security number or Medicare provider number.
18	This refers to hospitalization admission and discharge dates.

19	This item is left blank for local use. Contact the payer to determine their specific requirements. It is often used to list items such as which tests were administered.
20	This box is typically checked as *no* in mental health. It is used for payment of lab procedures conducted outside of the clinic. Check with the local payer for their requirements regarding Chemical Dependency urine lab results, lithium levels, and so on.
21	Enter the most current International Statistical Classification of Diseases and Related Health Problems or *DSM* code as required by the payer. Do not type in decimals.
22	For Medicaid claims only.
23	Enter the preauthorization number(s) from the payer.

Block 24	**Services Dates, Procedures, Services, Supplies**
24A	In the *From* column, enter the date of each service in the MM/DD/YYYY (or YY) format. In the *To* column (typically not used in mental health), enter the last date if the same procedure was performed on consecutive days. It is most common to bill for services day-to-day.
24B	Enter the *Place of Service* code, which is the place where services took place. Although several codes are not listed, the codes that could apply to mental health services are as follows

03   School
04   Homeless shelter
05   Indian Health Services, free-standing facility

06   Indian Health Services, provider-based facility
07   Tribal 638, free-standing facility
08   Tribal 638, provider-based facility
11   Office
12   Home
15   Mobile unit
20   Urgent care facility
21   Inpatient hospital
22   Outpatient hospital
23   Emergency room–Hospital
31   Skilled nursing facility
32   Nursing facility
33   Custodial care facility
34   Hospice
50   Federally qualified health center
51   Inpatient psychiatric facility
52   Psychiatric facility—Partial hospitalization
53   Community mental health center
54   Intermediate care facility for mentally retarded
55   Residential substance abuse treatment facility
56   Psychiatric residential treatment facility
99   Other unlisted facility

24C   Blank.

24D   Enter the CPT code and modifiers, if appropriate.

24E   Enter the Diagnosis Reference Number 1–4.

24F   Enter the fee for the service. There is space for up to six services per claim.

24G   Enter the number of units for the service. In mental health, most units are in 1-hour increments, but variation exists. Contact the payer to define the prescribed amount of time given per unit for each service.

24H	Blank. For Medicare claims only.
24I	Mark an *X* if the service was provided in a hospital emergency room.
24J	Blank, unless the client has secondary insurance, then mark *X*.
24K	Blank. For local use, if requested.

	Provider Information,
Blocks 25–33	**Charges for Services**
25	Enter the providers Employer Identification Number (EIN), and check the EIN box. If there is no EIN, write the SSN and check the SSN box.
26	Enter the account number you assigned the client, if any.
27	Check *yes* if you choose accept assignment. This means that you accept the amount that the payer pays. Check *no* if you are not a participating provider with the payer.
28	Enter the total amount of the claim, which is the total of the charges listed in Block 24F. Do not add the total amount of claims on other sheets.
29	Enter the total amount the client has paid to date toward the current yearly deductible, coinsurance, and co-payments.
30	This amount is the amount in Block 28 minus the amount in Block 29.
31	Enter the full name and professional credentials of the provider and the date in MM/DD/YYYY format.
32	If services were provided in a place other than the provider's office or the client's home, list the address where services were performed.

33   Enter the phone number, billing name, and mailing address. If you are a participating provider, enter the PIN and group numbers. If you are a nonparticipating provider leave these items blank under the address.

SUMMARY

Medical billing is a fairly complex task. There are multiple codes, rules, and knowledge requirements that if not known and followed, will lead to the rejection of claims. Information on the form must be filled out exactly how the third-party desires. Billing formats and acceptable codes may differ between third-party payers. Some payers require referrals, others require a prior authorization for services, while others allow you to see the client for a stated number of visits.

It is common that there must be an Axis I diagnosis if therapy takes place; however, some third-party payers do not provide payment for certain Axis I diagnoses. Therefore, the person at the clinic who conducts the billing is a very valuable resource.

There are times when insurance does not pay for services, such as when a deductible has not been met, when they are not the primary insurance company, or the charge is for a noncovered service. Also, many clients will not have insurance. Thus, it is important to have a binding contract for services that covers fees and provisions for payment.

When an insurance claim is rejected, do not give up. There are many possible reasons for the rejection. Sometimes, simply resubmitting the form results in payment. Clerical and scanning errors happen at insurance companies. Insurance rejection slips typically explain why a claim has been denied. Check their reason, and, if appropriate, rebill the claim when the error is corrected.

The CMS-1500 is the standard insurance claim form. Although it is fairly self-explanatory, those new to billing typically make several errors. There are billing programs on the market that make the task much easier.

TEST YOUR KNOWLEDGE

1. Most insurance companies do not pay for

    (a) marital therapy.

    (b) psychoeducational services.

    (c) Axis II disorders.

    (d) all of these.

2. Along with other demographic information, the payment contract should include

    (a) the Social Security number of the person responsible for payment.

    (b) the Social Security number of the client.

    (c) the diagnosis.

    (d) the name of the credit reporting agency.

3. Standardized policies and procedures for billing practices are necessary

    (a) only in large clinics.

    (b) only in accredited clinics.

    (c) at all clinics.

    (d) when therapists differ in billing policies.

4. A large reason many clinics experience financial difficulties is that

    (a) therapists are reluctant to ask for co-payments and deductibles.

    (b) there is not a payment contract.

    (c) they do not pursue denied insurance claims.

    (d) all of these.

Answers: 1. d; 2. a; 3. c; 4. d

9

Administrative, Clinical, and Safety Policies and Procedures

IMPORTANCE OF WRITTEN POLICIES AND PROCEDURES

Terms such as *policies and procedures* (P and Ps) are typically not very exciting to therapists. Far too many mental health professionals dislike rules and regulations, believing that they only lead to increased administrative time and paperwork. What many therapists are not aware of are the potential consequences of not having written P and Ps.

Policies are written statements describing the guidelines and principles the clinic has adopted for given situations. *Procedures* are the courses of action taken to follow a policy. For example, a clinic might have a policy to verify each client's insurance, prior to the first visit. The procedure might be (1) obtain the client's name, address, phone number, name of insurance carrier, policy number, and date of birth, (2) an assigned person phones the insurance company and verifies the insurance benefits, and (3) if covered, an assigned person fills out specific paperwork and notifies the therapist and the client.

Without this procedure, a client's insurance might not be verified, resulting in the clinic, therapist, and client possibly becoming upset regarding who is responsible for payment. Although a clinic should not have excessive policies and procedures, they should exist, especially in areas that affect client welfare, business practices, safety issues, and employment practices.

The larger the clinic, the more clear, well-written, agreed upon P and Ps are important. Even smaller clinics need consistent practices. Differences in or the nonexistence of standardized policies can only lead to miscommunication, disagreements, confusion, unequal treatment of clients and staff, and the appearance of a poorly managed clinic. Every employee and contractor in a clinic should be carefully trained and given a copy of the clinic's policies and procedures. Staff trainings should periodically review these practices. Although therapists who have never been exposed to such management techniques often resist this supposed breach of freedom, there will likely be an appreciation for such practices when a certain P and P brings order out of chaos in an emergency situation.

In addition to the examples of P and Ps in this chapter, clinic managers or directors must be aware of and comply with Health Insurance Portability and Accountability Act (HIPAA) regulations.

Example of Having P and Ps in Place

A client in the waiting room of a moderately sized outpatient mental health clinic yelled out, "I'm going to kill myself as soon as I get out of here." The only people who heard him were other clients in the waiting room and the receptionist. The people in the waiting room panicked. There were no therapists in the area because they were all in sessions with clients. The receptionist was not a mental health professional, but she had attended staff trainings that reviewed and role-played handling an array of clinic emergencies. She immediately followed a few steps in the P and P manual that led to team effort that quickly resulted in one therapist dealing with the client, while another therapist followed procedures to calm the people in the waiting room. At the same time, another employee handled a call to the hospital for medical transportation and made a call to the client's stated emergency contact.

Lesson: A receptionist without training might have panicked as did the clients in the waiting room. Such an action could have led to more confusion and increased problems and safety issues. However, prompt action, conducted by a well-trained staff, may have prevented a suicide.

Chapter 2 of my book, *The Clinical Documentation Sourcebook, 3rd ed.* from Wiley, provides a primer of HIPAA training.

The rest of the chapter will provide examples of several possible policies and procedures that could be helpful, depending on the size and nature of the clinic. Not all possible P and Ps are included, but a scope of possibilities is provided. They are divided into the following sections: (1) business, (2) clinical practice, and (3) safety. Discussions of selected P and Ps are covered in this chapter, and related examples are provided in the appendixes. The samples do not cover every possible P and P—those would comprise another volume—but provide a well-rounded sample. Individual clinics may have specific needs standardized P and Ps would not fit.

BUSINESS POLICIES AND PROCEDURES

Most of the business P and Ps have seemingly little to do with individual therapists, but they describe the nature of the business, plus its mission, structure, plans, finances, and safety procedures.

Business Plan

Few mental health clinics have a written business plan. It is clearly a business document dealing with fiscal matters, not mental health services. The business plan provides a reader detailed information and examples of the mission, background, leadership, structure, means of gaining business, staffing, income, expenses, goals, and potential risks of the business. An outside reader will carefully review the feasibility of the plan and compare its statements to other financial reports you provide. Therefore, be realistic and accurate.

Even if there is no outside source requesting a business plan, each clinic should periodically discuss each of these topics. A business has no clear direction without a plan. A business plan is based on empirical data from previous accomplishments and setbacks.

Established clinics write up a business plan when seeking accreditation. Some business plans are written prior to opening a business. The purpose is typically to secure a business loan. Important aspects of this type of plan include answering questions such as the following:

1. What services will be provided?
2. What is the level of need for this service?
3. Who are the potential clients?
4. Why will they come to your business?
5. Who is the competition?
6. How will you reach potential clients?
7. What physical and financial resources are available?
8. What are the start-up costs?
9. What reserve funds are available?
10. What are your goals for 6 months, 1 year, 2 years, and 5 years, and how will you realistically attain them?

The best business plans accomplish the following:

1. Hold the reader's attention.
2. Convince the reader that there is a ready market.
3. Clearly describe how current and future staff are capable of successful operations and growth.

Note: The Internet is replete with more elaborate sample business plans under key words such as *Business Plan Samples.*

Fiscal Management Policies and Procedures

Fiscal management policies and procedures help designate responsibility and provide accountability in the financial affairs of the clinic. As with several other P and Ps, a fiscal management policy increases in importance as more employees are hired. For example, if the business is a small private practice where the owner handles

Sample Business Plan

Description of the Company

_____ (name of practice) provides outpatient mental health services in _____ (geographical area the clinic serves). It was established by _____ (founder's name) in _____ (year). The governing business body of _____ (name of practice), in a board meeting held on _____ (date), approved _____ (name) as president and chief executive officer of the corporation. They approved _____ (name) as the clinical director. The clinic ownership is _____ (describe).

Their vision was to establish a comprehensive outpatient mental health and substance abuse clinic to meet the needs of the residents of _____ (geographic area the clinic serves). They wanted a facility where adults and children could be treated by a group of professionals who shared this vision and implemented this goal.

Note: In the next paragraph or two, describe any changes that have taken place in the direction, ownership, location, or any other important history of the practice.

Mission Statement

We, at _____ (name of practice), are dedicated professionals committed to providing quality mental health and substance abuse services. It is our overall goal to enhance the quality of life for individuals and families. Our belief is that all people are valuable and unique and should be treated with dignity and respect. While recognizing the potential for change, an assessment of the client's emotional, physical, spiritual, and life experience is provided in a caring environment. The growth of the individual is promoted through a course of treatment developed and executed in a timely and cost-effective manner.

Financial Forecast

In the year _____, net receipts for _____ (name of practice) were, $_____, of which $_____ was realized as profit.

Note: Describe financial strengths and weaknesses and what is being done about them. For example:

In an effort to control long-range costs, a number of changes have taken place that will benefit _____ (name of practice) financially after they are paid for. For example, at present, $_____ is spent yearly for billing services. This expense will be phased out beginning _____ (forecasted date) by the recent (lease or purchase) of a billing system (computers, software). The yearly lease price of less than $_____ (amount of new expense) will significantly decrease at the end of the 3-year payment period, during which only upgrade and maintenance expenses will be incurred. Initially, there will be an approximate $____ to $____ in yearly savings. There will be no need to hire additional staff.

Other changes have included the recent hiring of an intake coordinator. Prior to this hire, the intake system led to the loss of approximately 50 percent of all referrals to the clinic. Clients often waited several days to set up an appointment. At present, appointments are given immediately. This has resulted in increase of intakes, from 50 percent to 85 percent. The bulk of referrals lost at this time are due to an inability to file specific insurance claims. Due to this concern _____ (name of practice) has applied to three more insurance panels that were not used in the past and accounted for approximately 75 percent of the lost referrals. It is projected that the income from the increase in referrals will exceed $____.

Management Team and Key Personnel

Shareholders:

Note: Provide the names, degrees, titles, and responsibilities of the primary shareholders. Include a description of their professional backgrounds. Emphasize their experiences and abilities to manage a successful business.

Other management team members:

Note: Provide similar information, as in shareholders with specific emphasis on their responsibilities in the practice.

Advisory board members:

Note: Provide the names and a brief description of their type of work outside the clinic. Attempt to describe a board that represents a wide variety of perspectives from the community (e.g., mental health, schools, finance, minorities, religious, business, households). The board should not be one-sided, or be composed mainly of people directly related to, or employed by, the clinic.

Business Structure

_____ (legal name of practice) is incorporated under the laws of the state of ____ (name of state). The shares of the business are owned by _____ (names of major shareholders).

Marketing

_____ (name of practice) incorporates several means of making its services known. Internal research indicates that referral sources come from the following sources, in order of importance:

Note: List marketing strategies (e.g., previous referrals, fliers, contracts, The Yellow Pages, *signage).*

Each patient who phones the clinic for services is questioned as to the source of his or her referral. Marketing strategies are evaluated periodically and considered in the advertising budget.

With the competition for mental health services increasing, _____ (name of practice) avails itself of several opportunities to obtain referrals. We attend a number of community functions, sit on community board meetings, provide seminars for local schools, and regularly apply to be part of third-party payer panels.

The _____ (geographic area) area demographics continue to suggest both population and financial growth. _____ (geographic area) is rated in the top six counties in the _____ (region) in individual wealth. The residents of the area are highly educated, skilled, productive, and are a stable workforce. Several national corporations, including auto manufacturers, are located or have major offices in the area. The population dispersal of (home to the clinic) in _____ (year) was:

Age	%	Age	%
< 5	_____	30–39	_____
5–9	_____	40–49	_____
10–14	_____	50–59	_____
15–17	_____	60–69	_____
18–20	_____	70+	_____
21–24	_____		
25–29	_____	Mean age	_____

The median family income in _____ (year) in the _____ (geographic area) area was $_____. Surrounding communities' median incomes range from $_____ to over $_____.

Business Strategy

_____ (name of practice) will continue to expand its services, which match the needs of the community it serves. Needs are determined by the following methods:

1. Analysis of referrals' stated problems.
2. Attendance at community mental health meetings.
3. Analysis of response to marketing strategies.

As needs are identified, additional therapists are hired. For example, _____ recently expressed a need for a clinic with _____ (specific type of service) treatment for _____ (specific population). We are now working on an appropriate program, hiring new therapists, and writing a proposal to service the population.

Our advertising budget is substantial, regularly running over $_____ yearly, including radio commercials, advertising in several phone books, mailing-list fliers, and a web site. The return on our advertising budget is approximately X to 1.

Operations

The physical building of _____ (name of practice) is located in a prime real estate area. The nearby crossroads are well known to the community and conveniently located for public transportation. We currently rent over _____ square feet of space. The furniture and fixtures are kept in adequate condition and replaced as needed. We plan to stay in this location until at least _____ (date), when the lease expires.

Equipment

_____ (name of practice) recently (leased or purchased) a professional voice mail system. Previously messages were written. A live operator still answers the phone. Considerable clerical time is now saved and confidentiality in messages is preserved. The new billing system has provided the clinic with five networked computers.

Staffing

All staff members have job descriptions that are intended to eliminate redundancy. Clinical staff do not have to involve themselves in administrative duties unless they desire. Both clinical and office staff regularly attend training in safety and client issues. We have a staff of _____ clinical and _____ clerical members.

Forecast

Based on the improvements made in the year _____, the clinic projects a yearly receipt amount of $_____. The net profit is projected at $_____. We expect a steady buildup of clients due to (1) the increased percentage of referrals who receive services, (2) more contracts, (3) more services provided, and (4) recent increases in the fee schedule and in negotiated contract rates.

Income Statement

The yearly receipts since _____ (dated 5 years ago) have been as follows:

5 years ago	4 years ago	3 years ago	2 years ago	Past year
$_____	$_____	$_____	$_____	$_____

Profits

$_____	$_____	$_____	$_____	$_____

Expenses

The major nonfixed expenses of the clinic will be paid off in the next 3 years according to the current payment schedules. These expenses include the voice mail system, billing system, a bank loan, and payments to the previous owner. After these payments are eliminated, the yearly savings will be approximately $_____. Therefore, in the next few years no significant expenditures should take place.

Business Controls

The accounting system is computer based. With this system we review our income and expenses on at least a weekly basis. We analyze our profitability in every aspect of the clinic; thus, decisions to increase or eliminate programs are empirically based.

Capacity

Our offices accommodate _____ therapy and _____ administrative spaces. Therapy sessions last 1 hour, and the clinic is open _____ hours per week. Therefore, the capacity of the clinic is to see _____ × _____ = _____ clients per week if there were other offices available for nonclinical duties. If clients are available equally for each time of the day, the current office space is sufficient. Currently, the clinic averages 55 percent capacity. Growth can take place if more daytime hours are utilized by clients.

Long-Term Financial Goals

The financial objectives of _____ (name of practice) is to be debt free in the next 3 years. We anticipate steady growth and a profit increase of at least _____ percent per year. The purchase of a building is planned after bills are paid and a down payment is saved.

Steps for Achieving Goals

1. No significant expenditures for the next 3 years.

2. Caps on commissions received by new therapists.

3. Increased number of clients through the following:

    (a) more referrals

    (b) higher retention of referrals

    (c) increase services to community

    (d) increase types of service during non-prime hours

    (e) reputation of high quality services

    (f) increase clinical staff as needed

    (g) increase daytime services

4. Attempt to pay more than minimum on monthly debts.

Risks Associated with Growth

1. Decreased sense of personal touch due to clinic expansion.

2. Overextension of personnel.

3. Not being able to service demands of additional third-party payers' requirements.

4. Higher costs of larger building.

5. Increased competition with existing providers of services.

all finances, this set of P and Ps is not as important as in a larger setting, where decisions are made on a hierarchical basis. Nevertheless, even in a small clinic such policies, when followed, demonstrate accountability. For example, when the policy requires that an independent certified public accountant monitors the income and expenses, there is less chance of errors and fraudulent activity. When a clinic is being reviewed by entities such as accrediting agencies, certain third parties, the IRS, or a bank, evidence of financial accountability speaks volumes.

Sound fiscal management policies are not solely intended to prevent fraud. Careful monitoring of spending and income are necessary for budgeting, evaluation, and future planning.

In the written P and Ps, include who is responsible for purchases and describe their limits and when approval by others is required. Consider policies such as requiring two signatures for checks written by the clinic. Include approval of the board of directors for major purchases. Include a system of standardized clinic fees that can be revised only by the board. Avoid allowing one person to have excessive financial control. Clearly describe specific procedures regarding how clients are billed. Make clear policies and procedures about who receives payments from clients.

Describe the frequency and methods of how internal and external audits are handled. Describe how the results of financial reports will be incorporated. Overall, formulate a policy that creates shared accountability, with checks and balances of control.

Delinquent Accounts

Poorly organized clinics typically have no written collection policies in place. Less assertive therapists often expect that others will take care of collecting past due fees, or they let the fees go. Even when it is not necessarily the job of a clinician, this task is often ignored if it is not assigned to someone.

P and Ps must be in place to handle unpaid balances from clients. A clinic that waives insurance deductibles and co-payments will not stay in business very long or will have unnecessary financial

Sample Fiscal Management Policy and Procedures

_____ (name of practice) operates on a fiscal year of January 1 to December 31.

A formal budget of expenses and expected revenues is prepared annually, reviewed by the directors, and submitted for approval by the board of directors no later than mid-December of each year. A chart of accounts is maintained by the directors, which describes all expenses by category and all income by source. The Budget and Financial Statements shall conform with the approved Chart of Accounts.

Revisions in the budget exceeding a _____ percent variance in line items must be approved by the board. Variances of _____ percent or less may be approved by the directors.

_____ (name of practice) utilizes the services of an independent certified public accountant to regularly assist with monitoring expenses and income reports and to prepare all necessary reports and tax findings. Quarterly, a profit and loss statement, a cash flow report, and a balance sheet are submitted to the operating/quality assurance committee. Annually, the accountant prepares a compilation and review as the result of audit activities. This report is presented to the board of directors for review and to the shareholders at the annual shareholders meeting for evaluating stock.

An accounts payable system is maintained by the directors. All items in the accounts payable system are reviewed for conformity and authorization under the approved budget. Deviations require approval by the directors. Capital expenditures not preapproved in the budget and exceeding $_____ require the directors' approval.

A computerized check writing system is utilized. The computer system keeps track of all checks written. All expenses are allocated to categories conforming to the chart of accounts, as maintained for accounting and financial reporting purposes. All blank checks and the expense check ledger are maintained and secured in the director of finance's desk when they are not in use.

The director oversees the day-to-day operation of the facility. The facility manager supervises the storage of all supplies utilizing secure, closed storage closets. He or she, or a designee, does the necessary comparative shopping, supply ordering, and use monitoring. Reports of use are generated monthly, with the amount of expense included by department. These reports include special order and general supplies.

The operating/quality assurance committee reviews any major furniture or equipment purchases. Items that are needed, but unbudgeted and increase the relevant budget line item by more than _____ percent, are sent to the board of directors for approval. Items resulting in an increase of _____ percent or less per line item may be approved by the director or sent to the board at his or her discretion.

Testing and play therapy supplies and equipment are requested by the therapist requiring them. After approval by the director (or designee), they are ordered by the facility manager, or purchased by the therapist, who is then reimbursed upon presentation of a receipt for job-related activities.

Any out-of-pocket expenses for job-related activities by staff members may be reimbursed provided that the following conditions are met:

- Item has prior approval of the director(s).

- Item is authorized within the approved budget.

- An expense reimbursement voucher has been completed with appropriate receipts and signatures and submitted to the director(s).

All payments of expenses are made by checks. Signatories are approved by the board and filed with the bank and with any other financial institutions with whom _____ (name of practice) does business. Two signatures are required on each check. When a signatory leaves the corporation, new signature cards are filed immediately, and the change is approved by the board.

Purchases may be made under credit agreements only with approval of the director(s). Formal credit agreements are entered into only after the credit application and terms are reviewed by the director(s). Major credit applications and loans (over $_____) must be approved in advance by the board.

_____ (name of practice) activities are supported solely by fees for service and by payments from third-party benefit providers. A fee schedule is maintained by the director, which describes the customary charges for services offered by _____ (name of practice). The fee schedule is available to all personnel and clients.

Any changes in the fee schedule, or special provisions for a particular benefit program, must be reviewed by the operating/quality assurance committee and approved by the board.

Individual therapists may negotiate reduced service fees with individual clients when the situation warrants and at their own discretion. The administrative director must be notified of these negotiated arrangements, and a payment plan must be entered into in writing when appropriate.

All clients receiving service from _____ (name of practice) sign a fee agreement specifying the fee per session and the method of payment. The agreement specifies that delinquent accounts will be turned over for collection.

_____ (name of practice) maintains a policy and procedure for collection of delinquent accounts. Changes in this policy must be reviewed, commented upon, and approved by the executive committee.

No client accounts are turned over to collection without the approval of the primary therapist, following verification of account accuracy through billing and medical records. Prior to such action and with the approval of the therapist, written request-for-payment letters are sent to the client. When deemed advisable, the primary therapist may be asked to contact the client to negotiate a means of settling the account. Therapists have the following options at this point:

- Set up a new payment plan

- Recommend writing off the balance, subject to the Director(s)' approval

- Turn the account over to formal collection

If no payment is forthcoming and the account has not been written off, the account is turned over to _____ (name of agency) outside collections agency, which pursues collections.

Separate accounts are kept for all clients. Each account has a fee agreement and a separate computer record. The fee agreement is filed in the case record.

Each transaction (charge for service, payment for service, adjustments to accounts, collection activity, etc.) is entered into the computer by the administrative director or a designee. Input reflects the date, amount, type of transaction by code or statement, and any other necessary identifying information. Each therapist turns in a Charge Journal for his or her daily activities. Services indicated on these charge tickets are then posted to the appropriate client records. These tickets must indicate, at a minimum:

- Account number

- Service code

- Date of service

- Client name

- Type of payment

- Diagnosis

A daily therapist's journal is generated to verify the recording of all client service transactions. Each therapist is assigned a discreet computer number. Payments, adjustments, and services posted to the individual client records are listed on the daily therapist's journal and are maintained in billing records for 7 years.

As a secondary record, bank deposits and miscellaneous income are recorded in a monthly Income Journal by source and date. This journal is maintained by the finance director. Deposit records are maintained in carbon deposit ticket books by the finance director. Deposits are made daily (weather permitting) by the finance director or a designee. Checks arriving by mail or personally presented are stamped immediately with a *For Deposit Only* stamp and inscribed with _____ (name of practice), bank name, and account number.

Cash received is placed into an envelope listing the payer's name, the date, and amount of the payment, and the sealed envelope is placed into a locked area in the billing office. Cash and checks are placed in a *For Posting* envelope until the bank deposit is made. After posting, cash and checks are placed in a *For Deposit* envelope until the bank deposit is made.

No cash is kept in _____ (name of practice) aside from a petty cash fund, which is used on a discretionary basis by the director(s) or a designee. Petty cash in the amount of $_____ is kept and administered by the front office staff. A record of receipts and of all cash-outs is maintained for the petty cash account, with receipts required for cash-out transactions. The petty cash receipts are audited and reconciled each time the petty cash fund is replenished.

The director(s) maintains records on all dependent benefit payments, subcontractor insurance payments, and other internal financial transactions. At the end of the month, an internal audit of all financial systems is completed by the director(s) and the administrative director.

When the accountant reviews internal audit and financial reporting data and closes the books for the month, the following should be done:

- A printed check register is prepared for all bank accounts, and balances are reconciled.
- A detailed general ledger is generated by computer, with backup copies of all transactions updated daily and maintained off-site.
- Revenue and expense statement and balance sheet are prepared and reviewed by the board of directors at its next scheduled meeting.
- Any necessary tax forms are prepared for signatures and filed as appropriate.

- Issues, concerns, and other financial matters having impact on _____ (name of practice) operations are reviewed with the board of directors by the director(s) and by the external accounting service when appropriate.

Payroll is prepared on a fixed schedule, and all necessary payroll records are maintained. Payroll is the responsibility of the director(s). All employees are paid for work specified in their job descriptions, as verified by time sheets and other appropriate records. Employees are paid every _____ weeks for work performed through the pay period ending date.

Independent contractors are paid as specified in their work agreements, and verified by journal sheets or time sheets. Contractors are paid by the _____ day of each month for fees collected during the preceding month.

All payroll taxes are paid according to law.

All primary financial records are maintained for _____ years.

The director(s) is responsible for maintaining and monitoring all financial record systems. The administrative director is primarily responsible for maintaining and monitoring all financial information pertaining to client-related income and accounts receivable, under supervision of the director(s).

Following completion of such audits, results reported to _____ (name of practice) are reviewed by the board of directors. When deemed advisable by the board, responsive steps, actions or procedures that address particular audit results and findings are formulated by the board and referred to appropriate operating areas (including operating/quality assurance) for comment or implementation.

---

difficulties. Clinics should have specific P and Ps clearly understood by administrative and clinical personnel regarding how unpaid funds are collected. The following sample form is part of the P and Ps assigned to administrative and clinical personnel. Other forms (to follow) are provided to the clinic that coincide with these policies.

There is a common misconception in the field that a therapist cannot abandon the client if that client does not take care of financial obligations. This is clearly not the case. The payment contract with the client should clearly state that services can be discontinued due to nonpayment.

Sample Delinquent Accounts Policy

The primary therapist will advise the client when the account is delinquent. If no payment is received, there are two alternatives for the therapist:

1. Collect a payment at the next visit, or set up a specific payment plan:
   - Get a credit application from office.
   - Set up a credit plan with regular payments.
   - File payments with the billing office.
2. Meet with the billing assistant to arrange payment plan or other options:
   - Discuss payment options and responsibility with the client.
   - Inform client that you no longer intend to be his or her therapist, and explain why.
   - Detail to the client his or her condition, including problem areas, and encourage the client to seek help elsewhere.
   - If possible, provide names and addresses of other therapists or organizations where therapy may be received.
   - Cover these facts in your notes.
   - Consult with the director(s) or medical director to make sure you have considered all aspects of the case.
   - Send a letter to the client outlining the key points, and file a copy.
   - If the client threatens to sue you, notify the director(s) and your malpractice insurance carrier.

Write off all no-shows and determine if the bill should be sent to collections.

Sliding Fees

A sliding fee is a reduced fee a client pays, due to inability to pay the regular clinical fee. It allows people to receive services who may not be otherwise able to afford them. Typically, the fee is based on income and family size. That is, the lower the income and the higher the family size, the lower the fee. While some clinics ask for evidence of income and family size, others take the client's word. Some

Sliding Scale Fee Deductions for Clients without
Insurance and Who Cannot Afford the Usual Fee

The following numbers represent a percentage of the usual fee charged to clients who cannot afford services without such a waiver. For example, using the following table, if a client has a family annual income of $23,000, with 5 family members, the fee charged would be 60 percent of the usual fee. That is, if the usual fee is $100, then the client would be responsible for 60 percent of this fee, which is:

EXAMPLE   Income: $23,000 $100.00 (usual fee)

Dependents: 5   × .60 (60%, as per following chart)

$60.00 sliding scale amount

The following sliding scale fees may be given over the phone. Clients must supply proof of income to receive a sliding fee.

Family Size	Income (in thousands)							
	< $16	$16–21	$21–26	$26–31	$31–36	$36–41	$41–46	> $46
1	65%	70%	75%	80%	85%	90%	Full	Full
2	60%	65%	70%	75%	80%	85%	90%	Full
3–4	55%	60%	65%	70%	75%	80%	85%	Full
5+	50%	55%	60%	65%	70%	75%	80%	Full

clinics go beyond the income and family size requirements and request that the client provides other evidence they cannot afford services. In some clinics, where the therapist is paid on a commission, therapists are given the option whether to see sliding fee clients because both the clinic and the clinician will make less money. Some clinics require that therapists see a certain percentage of sliding scale clients. These variables are typically written in the therapist's contract.

It is especially important to clearly document that the sliding scale fee is the exception in the clinic, rather than the rule. This is important because if it is demonstrated that the average fee charged to clients in a clinic is significantly lower than that which is charged to an insurance company, the insurance company might have a case for claiming they are being overcharged.

If a clinic uses a sliding fee schedule, it should be standardized so it is not unfair to each person applying. That is, two people with the same financial situation should not be charged different fees. Clients should be treated equally and fairly in all matters.

Clinic Fee Schedule

A clinic fee schedule is the published rate charged for each service provided by the clinic. It is used across the board in areas such as federal disclosure laws and insurance billing and is the basis to determine sliding fees. If there are any exceptions to the published fees, they should be included or amended to the schedule. For example, different rates are charged for therapists based on their educational or licensure level. Some clinics also include higher fees for highly experienced therapists or reduced fees for interns. Each of these fees should be disclosed, in order that the client can make an informed choice.

For those not acquainted with insurance payment policies, insurance payment is based on set fees paid by the insurance company, not the fee charged by the clinic (unless the clinic charges less than what is paid by the insurance company).

Designated Authority

The designated authority document clearly describes the leadership and decision-making processes in the clinic. It describes when the board meets and what takes place in the meetings. The types of decisions designated to the board are listed. The responsibilities of others, such as the CEO, president, various governing committees, and therapists are clearly defined. The overall duties of those making major decisions for the clinic are integrated with the bylaws and mission of the clinic.

Example of a Clinic's Fee Schedule

Procedure	Code	Degree	Hourly Rate (45–50 min)
Initial interview	90801	Masters	$_____
		Doctoral	$_____
Extended	90808	Masters	$_____
		Doctoral	$_____
Half	90804	Masters	$_____
		Doctoral	$_____
Individual	90806	Masters	$_____
		Doctoral	$_____
Family w/ patient	90847	Masters	$_____
		Doctoral	$_____
Family w/o patient	90887	Masters	$_____
		Doctoral	$_____
Partner relationship—Half	97100	Masters	$_____
		Doctoral	$_____
Partner relationship—Full	97101	Masters	$_____
		Doctoral	$_____
Partner relationship—Extended	97102	Masters	$_____
		Doctorate	$_____
Group	90853	Masters	$_____
		Doctorate	$_____
Testing	96101	Masters	$_____
		Doctorate	$_____
	96102		$_____
	96103		$_____
Psychological evaluation	S9194	MD	$_____
Medication review	90862	MD	$_____

Sample Designated Authority Policy

Purpose

The board of directors of _____ (name of practice) has final responsibility for the overall operations of the facility. They insure accountable corporate functioning that adheres to the articles of incorporation, the bylaws, state licensure, accreditation standards; federal, state, and local standards, rules, and regulations; and other applicable standards and requirements.

Meetings

The board meets at least annually. Minutes of the meeting are kept and include the following:

- The date and time of the meeting
- The place of the meeting
- The names of the attendees
- Business discussed
- All actions taken or policies made
- Implementation dates where appropriate

Facility Ownership

_____ (name[s] of principal owner[s]) provide direction for the program.

Note: Provide additional names and titles if the ownership is not involved in the daily operations of the practice.

Board of Directors

Overall responsibility and authority for clinic operations rests with the board of directors. The board comprises elected shareholders of the corporation, its chairperson, and president (the corporation's principal shareholder). Other individuals may serve on an ad hoc basis, but shall not have a financial interest in the corporation, and shall not be eligible to vote on matters that come before the board. The board of directors of the clinic is responsible for establishing, reviewing, revising, and administering the policies of the clinic consistent with various third-party accrediting, licensing, and funding bodies, as well as applicable federal, state, and local law.

The board is responsible for development and communication of the mission and vision of the clinic. Through the president or CEO, the board develops policies and procedures and makes sufficient resources available to insure that the clinic is capable of providing appropriate and adequate service. By adopting a program to assess and improve the quality of care and to appropriately address identified problems or opportunities to improve, the board actively participates in the monitoring of all services provided. The following is intended to be an overview of the relationship of major board of director functions with the remainder of the leadership structure.

Policies and Procedures

The board of directors, through the president or CEO, develops policies and makes sufficient resources available to assure that the clinic is able to provide appropriate services to its patients.

The board of directors oversees the financial management system and its accountability. The board of directors makes sure that there is adequate insurance.

The board of directors adopts a program of quality improvement, as recommended by the governing body.

The board of directors develops a set of bylaws, rules, and regulations that clearly defines the relationship between the board of directors, the president or CEO, and the clinical staff.

The board of director's bylaws, policies, and procedures define how the board of directors, the administrative, and the clinical staff function together and participate in the development of policies and procedures.

The board of directors must approve the appointment and privileges of clinical staff as recommended by the executive committee.

The board of directors must approve all budgets and revisions to the budget.

The board of directors must approve the written plan for professional services.

The board of directors must approve the Continuous Quality Improvement, developed by the governing body Utilization Review (UR) Plan.

The board of directors must approve the personnel practice policies as developed by the administration.

The board of directors must approve policies regarding patients' rights.

With the exception of the board of directors bylaws, the administration and the clinical staff must develop policies and procedures that regulate their performance and duties. All clinic policies and procedures must be reviewed and approved on an annual basis by the board.

The board of directors should review CQI results quarterly.

The executive committee will develop goals and objectives annually that are in keeping with the mission and philosophy of the organization. The executive committee shall perform an annual evaluation of the entire program and report the results of the evaluation to the board of directors.

The governing body shall approve ethics policies and procedures that address the following issues:

- Communication of the program's ethical standard to each person served

- External communication about the program

- This communication may occur via brochures, application to managed care companies and third-party payers, licensing bodies, and the local health department

- Communication regarding persons served

All communication with outside sources will be conducted in such a manner as to be within the scope of the ethical standards adopted by the agency, as well as those set forth by the professions of psychology, psychiatry, counseling and social work, and shall follow all rules and laws governing confidentiality. Such communication may take the form of brochures, newsletters, and reports to referral sources.

The governing body of _____ (name of practice) will review ethical standards when the agency's policies and procedures manual undergoes annual review by the board or at such time during the course of business that a change in the ethical standards is deemed necessary.

Whenever a conflict of ethical behavior or recipient rights arises, the organization shall endeavor to resolve the issue in an ethical and expedient fashion. Questions of unethical conduct on the part of staff shall be referred to a peer supervisory process if all parties involved are in agreement. The intent of peer supervision is to fully evaluate the perceived breach of ethics and to counsel the staff member on a more appropriate approach. Peer supervision shall advise the administration of its findings and recommendations, as well as any resolutions to the problem. However, peer supervision shall not limit the administration from taking any corrective actions it deems necessary or preclude the staff member from the grievance process. Those staff members unwilling to engage in the peer supervision process may excuse themselves without prejudice, but the normal supervisory and grievance process shall take effect immediately. Gross misconduct shall result in immediate suspension of privileges until a formal hearing can be convened. Those staff persons found guilty of gross misconduct shall have all privileges and rights revoked in compliance with administrative rules and governing body bylaws.

Chief Executive Officer

The chief executive officer shall be a health professional with appropriate professional qualifications and experience, including previous administrative responsibilities in an outpatient psychiatric facility.

The chief executive officer shall have at least a master's degree in administration, psychology, counseling, or social work and, when required, should have appropriate licenses. Experience may be substituted for a professional degree if carefully evaluated, justified, and documented by the board of directors.

In accordance with the governing body bylaws, rules, and regulations, the chief executive officer shall be responsible to the board of directors for the overall operation of the organization, including the control, utilization, and conservation of its physical and financial assets and the recruitment and direction of staff.

The chief executive officer shall assist the governing body to formulate policy by preparing the following items:

- Long-term and short-term plans for the organization
- Reports on the nature and extent of funding and other available resources
- Reports describing the organization's operations
- Reports evaluating the efficiency and effectiveness of the organization's program activity
- Budgets and financial statements

The chief executive officer is responsible for the preparation of a written manual that defines organizational procedures and is regularly revised and updated. The operating and procedure manual, called the *Standards of Practice Manual*, of _____ (name of practice) shall contain the written policies and procedures required by _____ (accrediting agency, if applicable).

President/Chief Executive Officer

The president/CEO is responsible to the board of directors for the overall operation and direction of the organization through the powers delegated by the board. Routine responsibilities include the control, utilization, and conservation of physical and financial assets, and the recruitment and direction of staff. In collaboration with the executive committee, the president/CEO develops an annual budget and long-term capital expenditure plan.

The president/CEO is responsible for presenting this budget and plan (as well as regular reports relating to clinic performance) to the board for review and approval.

The president/CEO is responsible for the development of a comprehensive staffing plan. This plan, based on the needs of the individuals served and the clinic's goals and objectives, ensures availability of sufficient staff to adequately assess and address the identified clinical need of the population served and to coordinate the various services provided. When appropriately qualified clinical staff is not needed on a full-time basis, arrangements are made to obtain sufficient services on a consulting or part-time basis.

Governing Body/CQI Committee

The board has established a governing body/CQI committee, which is responsible for the leadership of the clinic. All policies, procedures, and reporting is forwarded to, or originated from, this board. The governing body/CQI committee reports directly to the board of directors, and is comprised of the president/clinical director, assistant clinical director, director of finance, and the director of development.

Executive Committee

The board has established an executive committee of the staff responsible for the monitoring and evaluation of client services and identification and resolution of problems concerning the performance of clinical staff and other clinicians providing clinical services. The executive committee is comprised of the president/CEO, the clinical director, the medical director, the director of finance, the director of development, the director of adolescent services, and the media director. Additional members may be added at the discretion of the CEO, as is warranted by additions of programs or services.

The board shall approve the policies and procedures governing the activities of the clinical staff. In addition, the president/CEO and the executive committee are responsible for establishing the process of designating clinical privileges, and shall include that process in the clinic's policies and procedures manual. The board of directors, through the executive committee, while following the clinical staff policies and procedures and the process of designating clinical privileges, shall ensure that services provided meet the standards for quality contained in the clinic's policies and procedures manual and that any failure to meet those standards is promptly corrected.

The executive committee has responsibility for the quality of all clinical care provided to clients and for the ethical and professional conduct of its members. The board grants the administrative and professional staff the authority and freedom to carry out their responsibilities within established policies and procedures. The executive committee shall measure patient involvement in care and feedback through the patient (via formal client satisfaction measures) as part of its efforts to improve clinic performance.

The executive committee shall ensure that each member of the clinical staff is qualified for practice and shall encourage the optimal level of professional performance of its members through the appointment and reappointment procedure, specific delineation of clinical privileges, and periodic reappraisal of each staff member. The president/CEO assigns clinical privileges upon recommendation of the executive committee. The board of directors has ultimate approval authority of all appointments, reappointments, and clinical privileges.

Specific Leadership Functions

The following policies and procedures specify the functions of the clinic's leadership in relationship to the following:

- Board of directors (bylaws)
- Clinical staff policies and procedures organizational evaluation
- Written plan for clinical services fiscal management
- Staff growth and development

It is our philosophy that all individuals have intrinsic value and that mental health problems can develop as a result of trauma, adjustment reactions, family dysfunction, and many other origins. By thoroughly assessing the client, these traumatic events can be identified, and the client can be taught to understand these events in a way that allows growth beyond the limitations imposed by the trauma. The client is able to gain insight and thereby take action to improve overall well-being. We provide both a traditional mental health approach to treatment and integrate cultural and spiritual perspectives for clients who desire such an orientation.

Substance abuse and addiction are progressive, chronic, and life-threatening diseases that are treatable. We believe that through education and an understanding of the disease a client can modify his or her behavior to live a healthy life. The client's independent functioning is strongly encouraged as he or she takes responsibility for recovery. We believe that an educated client will experience the fears, losses, passivity, and poor time structuring that crucially affect the early stages of recovery and, therefore, will be able to deal with these issues in a therapeutically successful manner. The client is encouraged and supported to experience and overcome these obstacles to recovery by using new and proven techniques.

We believe that people should be treated with professionalism, and we strive to always improve our care of the client. We believe that therapy does work and that we not only need to continue to be educated, but that we also need to arm our clients with education and empower them to move on. It is our goal to have integrity in all of our dealings. We not only have strong values ourselves, but also emphasize strong values in our clients.

It is our belief that all people should be treated with dignity and respect. Clients should be treated with the most appropriate level of care and in the least restrictive environment. We do not force any religious or spiritual approach in counseling, but have it available for anyone who needs or wants this aspect emphasized.

Goals and Objectives

Our primary goals are to improve our clients' quality of life by adjusting behavioral patterns, habits, and family relationship dynamics, and to develop insight into why these patterns develop, as well as what is required to develop healthy patterns.

Objectives for Mental Health Services

- To assess the client's current situation and develop a hypothesis as to how or why the current dysfunction is occurring

- To develop an understanding of why the client is experiencing dysfunction in his or her life, based upon the various biopsychosocial antecedents

- To help the client understand why he or she functions in a certain way

- To adequately plan for the client's recovery by integrating information from the assessment and then negotiating a comprehensive course of treatment

- To achieve a level of homeostasis where the client is comfortable and functional or to achieve a maximum level of function with expressed client satisfaction

- To develop a trusting relationship with the client so that they may develop an understanding of how to achieve the goal of mental health through healthy behavior

Objectives for Chemical Dependence Services

- To review and discuss issues of addiction and relapse
- To clarify the antecedents as events that occur prior to beginning chemical use
- To provide basic information on the progression of addictive diseases as well as information on recidivism and cross addiction
- To describe health problems and physical symptoms caused by abuse of alcohol and other drugs and to assist the client to personalize this information
- To increase awareness of dynamic patterns of behavior in the addicted person's family that leads to use and relapse
- To provide information regarding relapse and recovery and to encourage the client to choose recovery by developing a specific, active program of treatment
- To provide a supportive environment for the addicted person to explore and cognitively understand his or her abuse and addiction
- To provide a supportive environment for the codependent and enabling individuals to increase knowledge of specific roles in the addicted relationship
- To prepare and assist the client and the client's family in utilizing recovery support groups more effectively
- To provide the client and the client's family with an aftercare plan for continuing recovery

Accreditation
Accreditation processes are handled by the governing body, and any and all clinical, administrative, and support staff needed to assure that _____ (name of practice) remains in compliance with the standards of accreditation. If needed, the governing body can form an accreditation committee to coordinate accreditation processes and functions.

Closure of Clinic
The board of directors will retain sole authority for closing any clinic sites or programs. In such cases, the board, through the directors, will complete all appropriate forms and notify accrediting bodies and all other legal entities with whom the corporation does business, not less than 30 days before the closure of

any site or program. The board of directors will notify all therapists no less than 45 days before the closure of any site or program.

At this time, the Center for Substance Abuse Services and the coordinating agency will be notified. Clients will be referred to another licensed program or individual practitioners who are qualified to treat the clients.

Designated Authority, Advisory Board, and Staff List

Board of Directors

(Name and title of Board President)

Governing Body

(Names and titles of governing body)

Administrative Staff/Executive Committee

(Names and titles of executive committee)

Citizens' Advisory Board

(Names and titles of citizens' advisory board)

CLINICAL POLICIES

Policy for Interns

Both large and small practices typically make use of interns. A clinic can usually expect interns to have some counseling experience, but this is not always the case. It is the clinic's responsibility to determine the intern's level of competence and choose appropriate supervision, goals, and selection of clients. Interns should be scrutinized at the level of a beginning therapist. This includes a criminal background check, reference checks, and a thorough interview. They should have an appropriate level of liability insurance, which is typically covered by their college or university. Just as with any other employee, supply them with a job description, noting your expectations. In addition, clearly inform interns as to what they can expect from you.

Sample Policy for Interns

Interns are used in the following manner:

1. Each intern is assigned to an appropriately licensed and clinically credentialed mental health professional (e.g., psychologist, social worker, professional counselor, licensed marriage and family therapist) for supervision. They receive individual supervision at least once per week, plus group supervision, when available. The center provides supervision concordant with the regulations of the school the intern is attending (which are concordant with state regulations). Generally, counseling duties are increased as the intern's experience and competencies increase. Written evaluations are provided to the intern's respective school. Feedback is given after each observed session.

2. Interns are provided with a written job description. Job qualifications are equivalent to those of a beginning therapist, except for the graduate degree. This information is given during orientation, which is the same orientation received by a new therapist.

3. Interns must meet the same qualifications as a new therapist if they are to see clients independently. Beginning therapists do not see clients on their own without appropriate supervision (group observation, cocounseling) and approval of their supervisor. Interns must have the equivalent coursework qualifications of entry-level therapists. Practical counseling experience is developed through observation, case consultation, and supervised counseling. Interns do not see clients independently if fees are being paid by third-party payers. Clients are informed when the person providing services is an intern.

4. Interns are required to have a $1 to $3 million dollar insurance policy, which is the same requirement for clinicians at the center. Before interns can begin at the center, they are required to show proof of insurance. The intern's respective college or university generally covers the insurance needs of interns.

5. Interns, in their orientation session, are informed of the benefits and risks of their position. Topics such as confidentiality, liability, dealing with violent clients, and health and safety issues are covered in the clinical orientation. They also take part in clinical staff meetings that provide such training.

Ethics Policy

Every clinic needs a written ethics policy. This policy should be required reading and be signed by all staff as part of their employment contract. An ethics policy formally describes the clinic's dedication to ethical standards in all aspects of clinical and administrative practice. It further describes ethics violations as potential for termination and other professional and possible legal, consequences. Minimally, it contains references to the ethics of their licensure or credentialing source, plus any other provisions pertaining to specific ethical standards of the clinic.

Ethics statements primarily refer to a client's rights and quality of care procedures, as well as means of handling ethical complaints. Typically, a code of ethics is either given to each client, or it is clearly posted in the clinic.

Job Performance Evaluations

A job performance evaluation policy is designed to standardize the criteria by which different employees are evaluated. The information is used for retention, promotions, and pay raises. It is intended to provide employees with feedback to help increase their effectiveness. The policy is helpful in communicating when an employee can expect to be considered for a raise in pay. It delineates the time of the probationary period. It is intended to promote equal opportunities and fairness.

Staff Growth and Development

A progressive clinic provides the means for staff growth and development. This is typically obtained by in-service training for both administrative and clinical personnel. It is not uncommon for therapists to have a certain number of mandated training hours in their employment contract. Typically, a minimum number of training hours, either in-service or through continuing education

Sample Ethics Policy

_____ (name of practice) shall operate within the ethical standards set forth by the professions of psychology, psychiatry, counseling, marriage and family therapy, and social work.

In addition, _____ (name of practice) has adopted its own code of ethics under which staff members practice. _____ (name of practice) code of ethics is distributed to each staff member. Each staff member practices both within the ethical standards set forth by his or her own profession (psychology, psychiatry, counseling, or social work) and within the ethical standards adopted by the agency.

Each staff member is given a copy of _____ (name of practice) ethical standards, which they are required to review and understand. Each staff member is required to sign the agency's code of ethics, and this signed copy is placed in his or her personnel file.

Communication of the program's ethical standard to each client occurs during the client orientation process.

Each client is given a copy of _____ (name of practice) standards at orientation, along with the *Recipient Rights Brochure.*

The governance shall approve policies and procedures regarding ethics that address the following issues:

- Communication of the program's ethical standard to each person served.
- Communication of the program's ethical standard to each staff person.
- External communication about the program (This communication may occur via brochures, application to managed care companies and third-party payers, licensing bodies, and the local health department.)

It is the policy of the agency to provide a consistent and deliberate approach to ethical care and services within the community. We believe that all aspects of the business and care provided here should be influenced by our ethical guidelines.

The organization has several benchmarks that comprise our policy on ethical practices. These benchmarks are as follows:

- Clients should always be treated with respect, dignity, and the premise that they have intrinsic value as a person.
- Staff should always strive to satisfy the client with the services we provide.

- Staff should ask themselves if they treated the client with respect and if interactions were of a good moral character.

- Clients shall never be comprised or put into a situation that results in harm to them.

- The staff and organization shall always act in a manner that can be viewed as ethical and dignified.

- Clients will be treated in a professional and ethical manner that is consistent with the caregiver's professional code of ethics.

- The organization shall never engage in any behavior that would embarrass or appear improper to the community or other professional organizations.

- Quality shall be the core of our service delivery.

- Client rights shall always be observed and adhered to.

- Treat each person that interacts with the organization in a fashion that you would prefer to be treated.

The organization believes that all interactions with the community should be based upon an ethical framework that encompasses the spirit of community membership and citizenship.

The financial practices of the organization should be consistent with the guidelines outlined in the preceding. This does not preclude the organization from holding clients accountable for their financial obligations to the organization, but rather approaches the issue from a cooperative perspective whenever possible. We believe that we deliver a quality service at a fair price and expect to be paid for this service in a timely and fair manner. We attempt to educate our clients about their rights and responsibilities, including their financial responsibilities. We attempt to collect from insurance carriers whenever appropriate and make the client aware of financial obligations at intake. Whenever we are unable to collect from an insurance carrier, the client is billed for the services provided and is made fully aware that he or she is responsible for any charges not covered by insurance. Whenever the client disagrees with the billing charges, he or she has the right to discuss the account with the therapist, the office manager, or with a member of administration. Billing issues shall be resolved in a timely and caring fashion. Clients may be excluded from treatment due to their refusal to pay their accounts in a timely and appropriate fashion. Clients will be made aware of this policy as part of the intake process. Whenever a client is excluded from treatment as a result of nonpayment, they must be referred to another treatment provider to continue their care. Under no circumstance is a client to be abandoned as a result of nonpayment.

Our marketing practices are in keeping with the preceding guidelines and are very simple: "Only promise what we can reasonably expect to deliver and only provide quality service."

Conflicts of interest are to be avoided at all cost. The organization will not enter into any contractual arrangement where a clear conflict is present and would compromise the organization in any fashion. In the event a perceived conflict could occur, the governing body will be notified of the situation and their approval sought. If the conflict involves a member of the staff or a governing body member, they will be ineligible to vote on the issue.

Staff members of _____ (name of practice) are required to fulfill all the responsibilities of their job classification or appointment, in accordance with federal, state, and local laws; licensing regulations; professional standards; and center policy guidelines. Professional ethics require confidentiality of client information and the avoidance of sexual misconduct, substance abuse, and client mistreatment and abuse.

Whenever a conflict of ethical behavior or recipient rights arises, the organization shall endeavor to resolve it in an ethical and expedient fashion. Accusations of unethical conduct on the part of staff shall be referred to a peer supervisory process, if all parities involved are in agreement. The intent of peer supervision is to fully evaluate the perceived breach of ethics and to counsel the staff person on the more appropriate approach. Peer supervision shall advise the administration of its findings and recommendations, as well as any resolutions. However, peer supervision shall not limit the administration from taking any corrective actions it deems necessary or preclude the staff person from the grievance process. Those staff persons unwilling to engage in a peer supervision process may choose to do so without prejudice, but the normal supervisory and grievance process shall take effect immediately. Gross misconduct shall result in immediate suspension of privileges until a formal hearing can be convened. Those staff persons found guilty of gross misconduct shall have all privileges and rights revoked, in compliance with administrative rules and governing body bylaws.

Sample Job Performance Evaluation Policy

When an employee has successfully completed the 90-day probationary period, he or she will receive an evaluation of job performance. The decision to retain or dismiss the employee will then be made. A salary adjustment can be made at that time, according to the adopted salary scale in force. Thereafter, all performance evaluations will take place on an annual basis and will be done on the anniversary of the month of hire. This evaluation shall be performed by the immediate supervisor. At this time, the employee will be considered for an incremental increase in annual salary, the percentage amount of which shall be established by the director(s), but will be standardized for each position. There will also be periodic reviews of work performance to maintain the standards required by the center.

- Thereafter, any and all salary increases must be based on merit and job performance.

- While evaluation reviews may be required at various times, there will be no consideration of additional salary increases until the anniversary of the hire date occurs, and then only if there has been a successful written evaluation by the supervisor.

- All employee's evaluations, both 90-day and anniversary, must be completed within 10 working days of the end of the 90-day probationary period and subsequently on the employee's anniversary date.

- All evaluations shall, at a minimum, assess job performance in relation to expectations set forth in the job description, objectives established in the last evaluation, and objectives for the next evaluation period.

- Original signed copies of performance evaluations are located in the employee personnel files located in the locked file cabinet in the billing department.

(CE) opportunities outside of the clinic, are required. Provide ample time for new employees to learn the policies and procedures pertaining to their job. Typical in-service training covers topics such as safety procedures, crisis management, therapeutic techniques, documentation, and any number of administrative responsibilities. Many clinics allow time for staff training as part of a monthly staff meeting.

Sample Staff Growth and Development

Introduction

To increase quality of service, _____ (name of practice) encourages its staff to reach maximum potential in career development by providing training opportunities inside the program. Staff growth and development activities are under the direction of the executive committee; responsibility for the coordination of these activities lies with the clinic director/manager. The need for specific continuing education is identified through various activities. As problems are identified, one method of resolution may be attendance at continuing education sessions for one or more staff members. Additionally, individual staff members may request attendance at continuing education sessions that are particularly pertinent to an individual's area of treatment expertise or that he or she may wish to learn more about.

Documentation of attendance, with an evaluation of the training session, is completed by each staff member on the continuing education form. Completed forms are forwarded to the administrative coordinator for inclusion in the individual's human resource file.

In-Service Training

When in-service training sessions are held at the center, the clinic director/manager or a designee is responsible for completing the in-service training record and evaluation form. This form, as well as the continuing education form, and feedback received are used in the development of the annual evaluation of the staff growth and development program.

The clinic director/manager is responsible for including in-service training sessions for clerical and administrative staff in the overall staff growth and development plans. This plan is presented for approval to the executive committee to insure that planned services are in keeping with the findings of that committee.

New Staff Orientation

Orientation to the Center for new staff takes place on the new employee's first day. New employees are oriented to HR issues, including explanations of the fire plan and fire drills, particularly noting the plan for their own location. They are given a copy of the safety procedures with a signed receipt to be returned in 30 days, stating they have received and read the book. Safety and infection control procedures are reviewed. There is an orientation checklist that is filled out on this day.

The orientation also includes program safety and emergency procedures. Procedures are explained, including critical incident reports. The policy and procedure manual checklist is provided. This signed document is kept in the employee's HR File.

Staff Development Report
Reports of staff development activities are made in written minutes from the CEO to the executive committee. During the first quarter of the next fiscal year, the CEO or designee is responsible for completing an annual evaluation of all staff growth and development activities. This report, which includes evaluation results documented on the continuing education forms, is incorporated into the performance improvement annual report. Results of this evaluation are used when determining educational activities needed during the next year and any needed revisions to the staff growth and development program. An annual calendar will be developed at the beginning of the program year and will be reviewed and amended based on the quarterly reports.

As part of the biannual reapplication for clinical privileges, staff must have documented a minimum of _____ hours of continuing education. The _____ hours may be obtained at center sponsored in-services, or through attendance of external conferences, workshops, or by making a presentation at a workshop or conference. The administrative coordinator shall publish an annual list of upcoming center in-service training for review by all center staff. The administrative coordinator will keep a record of all in-services that staff have attended in their credential file.

Some clinics apply for CE credits for their staff training. This becomes a valuable benefit for employees because it saves them the cost of CE credits.

Clinics typically keep a log of the CE activities of therapists in their personnel files. When therapists receive their annual reviews, the staff development activities are used as part of the evaluation process.

Continuity of Care

Most clinics do not have the resources to take care of the needs of every client they serve. At times, services will be referred to other

Sample Continuity of Care Policy and Procedures

Referrals

Facility policy is to extend the client's continuity of care, whenever appropriate, by making referrals to resources that provide help or support that is beyond the mission or capabilities of the facility. Such services include examinations, assessments, consultation, special treatment services, and assistance from providers who can contribute to the client's well-being. It is also our policy to provide referrals and, where appropriate and possible, to provide a continuing flow of information concerning clients between the facility and the referral source, whether incoming or outgoing.

The services provided by _____ (name of practice), whether by staff or by referral, are coordinated to constitute an integrated program geared toward the accomplishment of the client's treatment goals and objectives. Therefore, all participants will keep in careful communication regarding the needs and progress of the client through the following means:

- A signed informed-consent form is always obtained prior to service.

- An assigned primary therapist coordinates all treatment service and is primarily responsible for communication with other service providers.

- All service providers are expected to provide input into assessment, treatment, and discharge plans.

- All service providers are responsible for preserving the client's dignity, safety, and human rights. The primary therapist is responsible for investigating and following up on any complaints of abuse, neglect, or rights violations.

- A record of all referrals is contained in the client's file; the record contains at least the following:

  - Place, date, and reason for referral

  - Contact person

  - Report of outcome, if available

- Appropriate releases of information are obtained from the client so that information may be exchanged freely between the facilities; this information includes at least the following:

  - Background information of the referral

  - Information on the client's treatment (i.e., current treatment, diagnostic assessments, and special requirements)

- Treatment objectives desired

- Suggestions for continued coordination between the referring and receiving resource

- Special clinical management requirements

- Information on how the patient can be returned to the referring facility

- The referring facility asks the referral resource to submit a follow-up report within a designated time period.

When making a referral, the state and federal rules of confidentiality are observed.

Incoming Referrals

Sources of referral include the following:

- Social agencies

- Hospital and other inpatient programs

- Physicians and clergy

- Business and industry (employers and unions)

- Court systems

- Spouses, family members, or other individuals

Written referrals may be documented through referral letters prepared by _____ (name of practice) or by the other agency. The receptionist logs all incoming referrals.

Outgoing Referrals

_____ (name of practice) maintains a written list of resources that are willing and able to provide services to the clients. This list contains sufficient detail to allow a staff member making a referral to determine the name and location of the resource, the types of services provided, and the eligibility criteria for service.

There is an updated directory of human service agencies for the county, which is kept in the business office. The directory is cross-indexed by human service need, and each listing provides the name of contact persons, addresses, and telephone numbers.

Continuity of Care

Whenever a therapist suspects or identifies a need in a client that seems to require specialized help beyond his or her, or the facility's, capabilities, the therapist should immediately consult with coworkers or a supervisor until sure of the proper procedure to pursue. Each client's needs are assessed upon intake according to the instructions in the assessment chapter of this manual. If the client has a personal physician, the client is directed to seek a physical assessment from that primary care physician.

Discharge Plan

Each client that enters treatment at _____ (name of practice) has a discharge plan prepared by the primary therapist. This document is part of a process that begins in the initial stages of treatment and is part of the individual plan. The discharge plan will serve to identify the client's need for another level of care and insure continuity of care. It is developed with the participation and input of the client. When appropriate, the client's family, legally authorized representatives, other appropriate personnel, or the referral source may be involved with the discharge planning process.

The discharge plan is maintained in the client's record and is referred to as needed to prepare the patient, as well as others (i.e., family, referral source, community agencies), for future discharge.

The discharge summary includes the following:

- Initial diagnostic impression (Axis I–V)

- Present diagnostic impressions

- Service and termination status (dates case opens and closes, overall client status at time of discharge, and reason for termination)

- Presenting problem and assessment (Why did client seek services, and what was the level of impairment? What are the client's strengths, needs, and abilities?)

- Clinical course (describes therapeutic interventions utilized in treatment, client's progress related to goals and objectives)

- Medical psychiatric status (summary of any psychiatric intervention the client received, a description of discharge medications, dosages, and instructions for use) Any referrals for further psychiatric care are documented in this section.

- Post termination plan (description of all aftercare referrals and recommendations) This includes the client's disposition and reaction toward the recommendations.

- Client's statement regarding satisfaction of treatment rendered (summary or direct quotes of the client's statements regarding satisfaction related to treatment process and discharge)

- Signed and dated by the primary therapist and the physician

The client who participates in the development of the discharge plan receives copies of the plan when appropriate. The discharge plan is maintained as part of the clinical record, and at no time shall a copy of the plan be released without authorization, per clinic policy.

Individual therapists, upon discharging a client, shall remain open to providing follow-up support when appropriately requested. The clinic will insure follow-up services to discharged clients through our *client satisfaction process*. This process occurs 90 days postdischarge and provides the client an opportunity to request further assistance, including referrals, and allows the clinic to receive data related to the effectiveness of treatment. Client confidentiality will be maintained per established state guidelines.

professionals. Policies regarding continuity of care cover areas such as client welfare, confidentiality, coordination of services, and communication between the clinic and the referral source. In addition, it covers provisions for aftercare in a discharge plan. It delineates specific procedures for the referral process. The policy also describes specific procedures and reasons for discharging a client.

Seclusion and Restraint

Sooner or later, depending on the nature of the clinic and clientele it serves, it is quite possible that a client will become out of control. Training staff to handle these emergencies is a must for any clinic. A policy is necessary to clearly instruct staff on the clinic's stand regarding seclusion and restraint of clients. Not having these procedures could lead to serious legal consequences.

Sample Seclusion and Restraint Policy

It is the policy of _____ (name of practice) that no staff member will practice the use of seclusion or restraint on any of our clients or their family members under any circumstances.

Our clinical staff is trained to avoid potentially dangerous situations with clients or their significant others. They are taught basic techniques to avoid situations when a therapist or a client could be injured, should someone become verbally or physically aggressive. Training also includes several techniques to escape situations involving physical confrontation with low risk of injury to either party.

Sample Recipient Rights Policies and Procedures

It shall also be the responsibility of the recipient rights officer to annually review these policies and procedures to consider necessary revisions. Documentation of this annual review and the majority approval of the governing body shall become part of the administrative record, as shall other pertinent findings of the recipient rights officer.

Specific Recipient Rights

1. A recipient shall not be denied appropriate services on the basis of race, color, national origin, sex, age, mental or physical handicap, marital status, sexual preference, or political or religious beliefs.

2. The admission of a recipient to this center, or the provision of prevention services, shall not result in the recipient being deprived of any rights, privileges, or benefits that are guaranteed to individuals by state or federal law or by the state or federal constitution.

3. A recipient may present grievances or suggest changes in program policies and services to the center staff, to governmental officials, or to another person within or outside the program without restraint.

4. A recipient has the right to review, copy, or receive a summary of his or her program record, unless the CEO or a designee judges such actions to be detrimental to the recipient or to others. Such a decision will be made if granting the request for disclosure will cause substantial harm to the relationship between the recipient and the center or hinder the center's ability to provide services in general.

If the director or a designee determines such actions will be detrimental, the recipient is allowed to review nondetrimental portions of the record or a summary of the record. If a recipient is denied the right to review all or part of his or her record, the reason for the denial shall be given to the recipient. An explanation of what portions of the record are detrimental, and for what reasons, shall be stated in the client record and signed by the CEO or a designee. All requests to review records will be directed to the CEO, who is the only staff member authorized to grant such requests and who shall identify the staff person to be present during the records' review.

5. A staff member shall not physically, mentally, or sexually abuse or neglect a recipient, as the terms "abuse" and "neglect" are defined in the Center for Substance Abuse Services licensing rules. "Recipient abuse" refers to either of the following:

- An intentional act by a staff member that inflicts physical injury upon a recipient or which results in sexual contact with a recipient.

- A communication made by a staff member to a recipient, the purpose of which is to curse, vilify, intimidate, degrade, or threaten a recipient with physical injury.

"Recipient neglect" refers to any incident that results in a recipient suffering injury, either temporarily or permanently, because the staff or other person responsible for the recipient's health or welfare was found to be negligent.

6. A recipient has the right to review our written fee schedule. Any revisions of fees will be approved by the governing body and all recipients will be notified at least 2 weeks in advance.

7. A recipient is entitled to receive an explanation of his or her bill upon request, regardless of the source of payment.

8. Should this program engage in any experimental or research procedure, any and all participating recipients will be advised as to the procedures to be used, and have the right to refuse participation without jeopardizing their current services. State and federal rules and regulations concerning research involving human subjects will be reviewed and followed.

9. The center does not engage in any research project which would involve behavior modification that uses painful stimuli, psychosurgery, electroconvulsive therapy, or any form of convulsive therapy. Nor does the center ever expect to engage in any of these treatment modalities.

10. A recipient shall participate in the development of the treatment plan. Counseling staff will inform recipients that development of a treatment plan is a cooperative effort between the therapy staff and the client. It is our policy that both the client and the therapist sign the master treatment plan, and any major revisions of that plan. Minor revisions do not require the client's signature.

11. A client has the right to refuse treatment and to be informed of the consequences of that refusal when it prevents the program from providing service. According to ethical and professional standards, the relationship with the recipient may be terminated upon reasonable notice. Reasons for termination will be recorded in the client's case file and in the discharge summary.

12. Upon admission each client is provided with program rules in the form of a treatment contract or a separate rule sheet. These rules are also posted in a public place within the Center. These program rules inform new clients of infractions that can lead to discharge. The rules also describe the mechanism for appealing a discharge decision, and which staff have authority to discharge. The client signs a form documenting that a written copy of the program rules were received, and questions regarding them were answered. This form is maintained in the client's file. Whenever appropriate, the length of time between discharge and readmission will be documented in the discharge summary, and discussed with the client.

13. A recipient shall have the benefit, side effects, and risks associated with the use of any medications fully explained to him or her in a language that they can understand. The medical director or consulting physician is responsible for providing this explanation, or for designating staff to do so. All clients receiving medications that have substantial associated risks will be asked to sign an informed consent form for that medication. (See appropriate policies and procedures.)

14. A recipient has the right to give prior informed consent, consistent with the federal confidentiality regulations, for the use and future disposition of products of special observation and audio/visual techniques, such as one-way mirrors, tape recorders, television, movies, or photographs. In the event that such devices or techniques are used, the client, therapist, and CEO or a designee will be in agreement as to the intended use and distribution.

15. Fingerprints may be taken and used in connection with treatment or research, or to determine the name of a recipient, only if expressed written consent has been obtained from the recipient. Fingerprints are kept as a separate part of the record, and shall be destroyed or returned to the recipient when the

fingerprints are no longer essential to treatment or research. However, it is not currently the policy of the agency to collect or use fingerprints.

16. These policies and procedures are provided to each member of the center staff. Each staff member shall review this material and sign a form that indicates he or she understands, and shall abide by, the centers' recipient rights policies and procedures. A copy of the signed form will be maintained in the staff member's personnel or credential file, and a second copy will be retained by the staff member.

17. The director shall designate one staff member to function as the centers' rights advisor. The rights advisor shall:

- Receive and investigate all recipient rights complaints without interference or reprisal from the program administrator.

- Communicate directly with the coordinating agency rights advisor when necessary.

18. The staff member designated as rights advisor shall not be a provider of therapy services, where staffing permits. In the case staffing patterns or expertise do not permit, the rights advisor will be assigned to review only cases that they have not been directly involved in.

19. Rights of recipients are displayed in a public place, or on a poster to be provided by CSAS. The poster will indicate the designated rights advisor's name and telephone number, and the regional rights consultant's name, address, and phone number.

20. As part of the intake or admission process, each recipient will receive a brochure that summarizes the recipient's rights.

21. It is the responsibility of the therapist to explain each right listed on the brochure to the recipient. The recipient will then be requested to sign the rights acknowledgment form or treatment contract, to indicate understanding. If he or she refuses to sign, then the refusal and reason given will be noted in the client's file by the therapist.

22. If the recipient is incapacitated, he or she shall be presented with the aforementioned brochure, explanation of rights, and opportunity to document understanding of the rights as soon as feasible, but not more than 72 hours after admission.

23. The procedure to be followed when the rights advisor receives a formal complaint is described in detail in the recipient rights procedure manual. It is

the center's policy that the center's rights advisor shall follow the procedures outlined in that manual.

24. Informal complaints, unusual incidents, and injury reports are handled on an individual basis by the center's staff.

25. In no way shall these rights and responsibilities limit the rights guaranteed to clients under law.

26. It is the policy of this center to respect the rights and dignity of our clients, and to have fully informed clients as our partners in the treatment process.

27. Whenever there is a question as to the rights of the client, it is our policy to error on the side of the client and to provide an ethical resolution of the issue. Clients may access the CEO to discuss any ethical concerns they may have.

28. Clients are always referred to the most appropriate level of care when clinically indicated and shall be seen at the least restrictive level of care. Likewise, the client shall be referred to appropriate external sources for services that the center does not provide directly. Therapists may access the referral book, or may consult with their supervisor or other colleagues to secure an appropriate referral for the client. Clients are referred to alternative services whenever they request.

29. Clients are entitled to adequate and humane services regardless of sources of financial support. This does not negate the client's responsibility to pay for the services rendered.

30. Children over the age of 12 will be involved in their treatment planning process at a level that is appropriate for their maturity level.

31. Appropriate staff are provided to clients based upon therapist expertise and availability.

32. Each client has the right to have an outside consultant review the treatment plan and give their opinion of the treatment plan. The cost of such a consultant is the responsibility of the client.

33. Clients who do not speak English as their primary language may secure the services of an interpreter if they wish to utilize the services of the center. Whenever the services of another facility would benefit the client more, the staff shall endeavor to refer the client to this facility. Some of our staff speak a second language, and a master list of therapists and their language skills are maintained by the administration.

34. Clients who are hearing or visually impaired may utilize the service of the center if their needs can be met within the confines of the program, with reasonable accommodation, as defined by the CEO or a designee.

35. The facility is physically handicapped accessible for those persons able to ambulate with either crutches or a wheelchair.

36. The program accepts only voluntary clients. Whenever a client is admitted to the program under a court order, the limitations of their rights, as outlined by the court order, are explained to the client by the therapist. Clients are referred to their attorney for the specific details of the legality of the limitations of rights regarding the release of information. The criminal justice release of information will be used for those clients who are under a court order, and require an exchange of information between the agency and the court.

37. Clients are informed of the clinic's responsibility to seek their commitment in the event that the client represents harm to themselves or others, or is unable to care for basic personal needs.

38. Clients are given itemized statements of their bill whenever possible. Charges for this service will be explained to the client. Clients are informed of any limitations placed upon their treatment by external sources and payers, whenever the center is aware of these limitations.

39. Clients are informed of conduct rules in the treatment contract and agree to abide by these rules while in treatment.

40. In the event that changes in clinical staff must occur, the client is informed of the reason for the change, and has input into new therapist assignments.

41. Clients are referred to appropriate aftercare and follow-up care, when appropriate.

42. It is the policy of the center to not withhold resuscitative services. We value human life and therefore will always call 911 (emergency services), per the center's policy and procedures.

43. In the event a client alleges abuse or neglect by a staff member, the CEO and the recipient rights advisor will be notified immediately. The complaint will be investigated, and the client will be informed of the outcome of the investigation.

44. If a staff person is found to be guilty of abuse or neglect, the client will be encouraged to file a formal complaint with the appropriate licensing body, and the staff member's privileges will be suspended until the end of the formal

licensing hearing. If the charges are found to be unsubstantiated, the client will be informed of the findings and no further action will be taken by the center. The client may appeal the decision of the CEO or the rights advisor to the governing body, or to the regional rights advisor.

45. Clients are not allowed to work for the center in any fashion. In the event that special circumstances should arise, and a client is allowed to work for the center, they will be paid according to the current wage scale associated with the job they perform.

46. Clients will always be treated with respect and dignity. It is our belief that it is unethical to harm clients in any way, and that to impede their right to treatment and good health is grounds for dismissal or revocation of privileges.

47. Whenever appropriate, family members or significant others of the client will be informed of how their involvement in the client's treatment could be beneficial. Whenever a client is unable to make decisions for themselves, family members or legal guardians will be consulted concerning the care provided to the client. If a conflict arises between the client and the family, the therapist shall seek consultation from a supervisor, the CEO or a designee. The supervisor may act as a mediator to assist the client and family resolve their disagreement.

Quality and Appropriateness of Services Authority

Every mental health practice or clinic should have some form of internal review of the quality and appropriateness of services. Even if there are no third-party auditors, or others to review files, it is always in the professional interest of the therapists and clinic to receive a professional opinion of the clinical documentation of ongoing services. These procedures help the clinic stay on track ensuring appropriate and timely services.

Typically a utilization review (UR) committee (several titles for the committee are possible) meets on a regular basis to review charts. They are given specific guidelines by clinic management or third-party sources. Depending on the clinic structure a number of methods of utilization are possible.

Clients are taught adaptive skills that are intended to generalize into other domains in their lives. Thus, additional functional impairments can be reduced or alleviated.

Sample Quality and Appropriateness of Services Authority

The executive committee and the governing body approved the utilization review (UR) and management plan of _____ (name of practice).

Scope

The utilization and management structure has been developed as part of the performance improvement program. The UR process will concentrate on appropriateness of admission, continued stay and discharge, as well as over and under utilization of resources. Resources are defined as people, space, money, and services delivered within the organization. Inclusive within this process is the establishment of a normal length of stay based upon internal data analysis and analysis comparative to external databases.

Objectives

The three objectives of the utilization review and management plan are to:

- Maintain and encourage quality care at _____ (name of practice).
- Ensure that care is being delivered in a responsible and efficient way.
- Ensure that resources are well managed.

Meetings

The UR committee will meet on a quarterly basis.

Conflict of Interest Statement

No UR committee member shall be given the responsibility or authority for reviewing his or her own records.

Methods of Evaluation

The two most common types of UR are *concurrent* review and *retrospective* review. Both elements are intended to improve the overall operation of the organization.

Concurrent reviews will focus upon open case reviews, and will be conducted to determine the relevancy of care for individual clients, as well as all clients being treated.

Retrospective reviews focus on closed records and determine whether clients receive quality treatment, evaluate outcomes of care, and identify patterns and trends of care that could effect operations and mechanisms of overall care.

There are three formal levels of UR:

- The consulting psychiatrist reviews all cases to determine appropriateness of admission, approve treatment plans, approve therapeutic assignments, approve the diagnosis, and approve continued stay and discharge.
- The peer utilization review committee (PURC) will review a sample of cases to determine appropriateness of admission, continued stay, and discharge. This committee will also review other key elements of care to determine if quality clinical care is provided, and to develop provider profiles. There is also a psychiatric peer review process.
- In those cases where the psychiatrists, the PURC or the medical records auditor question any aspect of care, the case will be referred to the utilization review team (UR team) for review and determination of care. The UR team is composed of the psychiatrist, a Masters of Social Work, and a fully licensed, doctoral level psychologist.

If the psychiatrist, the medical records auditor, or the PURC believe that a UR problem exists, they are charged to discuss the case with the clinician to resolve the problem or take the issue to the UR team for further review and a decision. The intent is to provide the appropriate service at the right time, in the correct intensity, for the correct duration.

Process of Evaluation
The following describes the process of UR at _____ (name of practice).

Psychiatric Review
The consulting psychiatrist reviews all cases to determine appropriateness of admission, approve the treatment plans, approve therapeutic assignments, approve the diagnosis, and approve continued stay and discharge. If he or she should question the validity of any of these elements, he or she will document the concern, and direct the therapist to conference the case or refer the case to the UR team for further review and disposition. The initial review will be within 10 days of admission, and at least quarterly thereafter to determine appropriateness of continued stay. The psychiatrist must approve all discharges 15 to 30 days prior to the actual discharge.

Peer Utilization Review Committee (PURC) and Psychiatric Peer Review
The PURC is composed of the administrator, a group of privileged clinicians that represent all disciplines, and the administrative coordinator.

The PURC will review a _____ percent sample of open cases to determine appropriateness of admission, continued stay, and _____ percent of all discharges. This committee will also review other key elements of care to determine if good clinical care is provided. Other elements include the effectiveness of assessment, the ability of staff to adequately document the care that occurs, timeliness, comprehensiveness, and effectiveness of clinical documentation.

The cases to be reviewed are selected by the administrative coordinator, who stratifies the sample by therapist. The cases are assigned to a clinician on the PURC to review who has not had any involvement in the case. The cases are reviewed prior to the monthly PURC meeting. The entire committee will discuss any case which has resulted in a negative response on the review sheet at the meeting. Any question of appropriateness of admission, continued stay, or discharge will be discussed and a decision will be made whether the case should be closed. PURC meetings will concentrate on specific elements per the review sheets.

The PURC will meet monthly, and information regarding patterns and trends will be aggregated and analyzed at least quarterly. The cases reviewed by this committee will be analyzed at least annually to determine long-term trend analysis, and to determine effectiveness of what and how we examine care delivery systems. One element of PURC is to develop provider profiles that will assist in the reprivileging process.

To determine that psychiatric care is being provided in an effective and efficient manner, a psychiatric peer review function occurs at least quarterly. A consulting psychiatrist will review the medical director's psychiatric evaluations and medication management practices to determine if consumers are receiving appropriate diagnoses, that medication prescribing practices are consistent with professional standards, and that medications are being prescribed in a safe and effective manner. It is the responsibility of the administrator to aggregate and analyze the findings of the consulting psychiatrist, and report this information to the PURC and the executive committee.

Utilization Review (UR) Team
The UR team is composed of a psychiatrist, an MSW, and a doctoral level psychologist. It is the final review process designed to provide direction to clinicians who question whether a case was appropriate for admission, continued stay, or discharge. In those cases where either the psychiatrist, the PURC, or the medical records auditor questions any aspect of care, and the questions are not resolved at a lower level, the case will be referred to the UR team for review and determination of care.

When a case is determined to be inappropriate for care or continued stay by the committee, the clinician will be notified to close the case within a specified number of days. The administrative coordinator will be asked to bring the discharged case to the next meeting for confirmation. If the case is not discharged, or the clinician feels that the case should remain open, they may petition the UR team to be heard. The clinician may appeal any decision for final review. Those clinicians who do not respond to the UR directive to close the case will be reported to the CEO, who may suspend their privileges.

The UR team will meet at least monthly and will aggregate the results of the review quarterly. Pattern and trend analysis will be developed based upon the aggregated analysis.

Retrospective Studies

While numerous elements could be studied, the most critical elements appear to be length of stay and outcome of impairments. Outcome studies include the measure of the length of stay across all diagnostic groups, by specific diagnostic groups, and by provider. This measurement and analysis allows administration to learn how well care is being managed in relation to the type of diagnosis, the provider, and compared to other outpatient centers.

Other measurements of UR include the timeliness, comprehensiveness, and effectiveness of record keeping as measured by the monthly internal medical record review and the biannual external medical record review. The review of space allocation is analyzed at least twice yearly, and the utilization and sufficiency of staffing patterns related to the timeliness of intakes is analyzed at least twice per year. All of these measurements are examined as part of our PI measurement process.

The second retrospective study is related to efficacy of discharge. It is important to know outside referrals that are made are appropriate and helpful to our clients. Referrals to inpatient and day-treatment hospital programs must be effective under the core function continuum. The center interviews at least a 25 percent sample of clients who are referred to the hospital, and aggregate the data from the following questions:

- Was the referral appropriate?
- Did the referral meet your need?
- Were you treated with respect?
- How was your relationship with the physician?
- Comment sections will also be available for additional remarks.

Hospitalization can be a traumatic experience, and we believe that aggregation and study of this collected data will increase our knowledge base related to the quality of care in local hospital programs.

Reporting of Information
Each of the two committees (PURC and UR team) will keep minutes of their meetings to be reported at least quarterly to the executive committee, and to the governing body. It is the responsibility of the administrator to collect and analyze the results of the psychiatric peer review process to the PURC and UR team, and ultimately to the executive committee.

Use of Information
The intention of the UR plan is to identify practice patterns, both positive and negative, and to use the data collected to make decisions regarding the improvement of care and operations at _____ (name of practice). We want to ensure consumers receive effective, efficient, and necessary care at the correct time and by the correct provider.

Summary of Utilization and Management Structure
It is our intention to provide high-quality care in a cost-effective manner. We will ensure that consumers who need care will have access to it, and that those consumers who do not need care, or have reached a level where care is no longer necessary, are discharged in a professional manner.

We believe that by following our PI and UR plans we can improve the care and operations of _____ (name of practice). Our goal is to implement these plans in an effective and efficient way.

Clinic Operations
_____ (name of practice) outpatient program (OP) is a traditional outpatient program that runs 6 days per week. The hours of the operation are Monday through Friday 9:00 A.M. to 9:00 P.M., and Saturday 9:00 A.M. to 5:00 P.M.

The population served includes all ages. The primary group being served is the population of the tri-county area, and the population of the geographic area consists primarily of middle-income clients. The clinic serves a significant adolescent population with primary referrals coming from area schools. Most of the substance abuse clients are referred from _____ (geographic area). Clients from all age groups come from our two primary referral sources, the radio program, and phone book advertisements.

Assumptions

The following information is based upon information from the National Institute of Mental Health, National Institute on Alcohol Abuse and Alcoholism, National Institute on Drug Abuse, and the Centers for Disease Control. It is our assumption that national statistics and trends can be extrapolated to a local level, and therefore can be assumed to be valid.

Approximately 18 percent of the general population is in need of mental health treatment, or can be classified as mentally ill at some level. Using these numbers one can estimate that of the 3 million people (according to the 1990 census) living in the primary market area, 540,000 are in need of mental health treatment. The number seeking treatment will vary from 20 to 35 percent of the total who need treatment. Therefore, conservatively, 108,000 people in the area are expected to seek treatment for mental health problems.

Approximately 10 to 15 percent of the general population is addicted to alcohol and other drugs. This can mean that in an estimated population of 3 million people in the primary market area, 300,000 to 450,000 people are addicted. The number of people seeking treatment will be approximately 20 percent of the total number who are addicted; therefore, 60,000 to 90,000 people will seek treatment.

The total number of people who are expected to seek either mental health or chemical dependence treatment is estimated at 168,000, conservatively. This number represents those individuals who make up the population we wish to serve. While there is no way to calculate for level of care, we believe these numbers are sufficient for justification of our services, especially since outpatient care is becoming the primary level of care in this area.

The primary market area is _____ (geographic area covered by the practice or clinic).

Admission Criteria

The program follows the admission criteria outlined in the most recent version of the *DSM* for mental health and substance abuse clients, and follows the basic admission guidelines for outpatients, as outlined in National Association of Addiction Treatment Providers standards. The program has also identified the following as other guidelines that define admission criteria.

- The client must meet the diagnostic category for mental health diagnosis as outlined in the *DSM,* and not be in need of a more intensive level of care.

- The level of impairment or dysfunction must impact the client's life in such a way that treatment is considered medically necessary.

- The client must be at least 3 years old, and have the approval of a parent or legal guardian to be treated. Family participation is required in the treatment of children.

- The client may not be actively suicidal or homicidal with specific plans for suicide or homicide. This would indicate a more intensive level of care is needed.

- Adolescents and adults (14 years and older) who are chemically dependent must have completed detoxification as necessary. Each client will have a history and physical screening form reviewed by a physician at the time of admission, and will be medically stable and able to engage in the program. The client will release the necessary medical records to the program to confirm the above. Other specific regulations may apply to third-party payers, per their requirements.

- Individuals must be motivated with sufficient internal and external resources to maintain a commitment to treatment, and be willing to enter into a treatment contract.

- The individual must have adequate support from family or a significant other who is willing to participate in the program with the individual, as required by the therapist.

- Addiction patients must be willing to commit to regular attendance at support groups in the community in addition to their OP involvement (e.g., Alcoholics Anonymous, Narcotics Anonymous, Alanon, Naranon) as appropriate.

- Client must not be in need of a more intensive or less intensive level of care.

Once the intake interview is completed and the client is determined to be appropriate for the program, he or she will be admitted to the program and will be oriented to the program rules and regulations by the therapist. Those clients not appropriate for the outpatient treatment are referred to other programs that may better meet their needs or required level of care. The office has a resource file available to assist with this referral or can send the client to community services for referral.

Program Goal

The primary goals are to positively modify the behavioral patterns, habits, and family and relationship dynamics, and to develop insight into why or how these patterns develop, as well as what is required to develop healthy patterns.

Mental Health Program Objectives:

- To assess the current situation and develop a hypothesis as to why or how the dysfunction is occurring, based on what has occurred in the past. This information is gathered through the comprehensive assessment and the *DSM-IV* criteria for mental health diagnosis.

- To develop an understanding of why or how the client is experiencing dysfunction in their life based on various biopsychosocial incidents. This information is gathered in the biopsychosocial information gathering in the initial sessions.

- To adequately plan for the client's recovery by integrating the information from the comprehensive assessment with the individual treatment plan.

- To achieve a level of homeostasis where the client is comfortable and functional, or to achieve a maximum level of functioning. This information is verified by outcome measures such as Global Assessment of Function, client satisfaction surveys, and commercial outcomes indices (e.g., Behavior and Symptom Identification Scale 32). Plus, the diagnostic criteria of the *DSM-IV* for symptoms and impairments must be decreased to a point treatment is no longer medically necessary.

Substance Abuse Program Objectives:

- To review and discuss issues of addiction and relapse. Clarify the antecedents as being events that occur prior to beginning chemical use. This information is gathered in the comprehensive assessment, including the biopsychosocial information.

- To provide information on the progression of the addictive diseases, as well as information on recidivism and cross addiction.

- To describe health problems and physical symptoms caused by the abuse of alcohol and other drugs, and to assist the client to personalize this information.

- To increase awareness of the dynamic patterns of behavior in the addicted person's family that leads to use and relapse.

- To provide information regarding relapse and recovery, and to encourage the client to choose recovery by developing a specific, active plan of recovery. This information is integrated in the individual treatment plan.

- To provide a supportive environment for the addicted person to explore and cognitively understand their abuse and addiction.

- To provide a supportive environment for the codependent and enabling individuals to increase knowledge of their role in the addicted relationship.

- To provide the client and family with an aftercare plan for continuing recovery.

- Overall, to achieve a level of homeostasis where the client is comfortable and functional, or to achieve a maximum level of functioning. This information is verified by outcome measures such as GAF, client satisfaction surveys, and commercial outcome indices (e.g., BASIS 32). Plus, the diagnostic criteria of the *DSM-IV* for symptoms and impairments must be decreased to a point treatment is no longer medically necessary.

Special Populations

The needs of special populations are identified through a number of means, such as the initial referral prior to meeting the client, at the initial meeting of the client, or after certain information has been disclosed in the initial screening.

The building at the center is handicapped accessible for clients with wheelchairs. If a client with auditory challenges desires services, a list of service providers with interpretive services is available at the front office.

The center credentials therapists to provide services to clients with various therapeutic issues and with various modes of therapy. The intake coordinator maintains a list of therapist competencies to assure an appropriate match. If there is not an appropriate match, or if a therapist is not available in a timely manner, an outside referral is given from a list of referral sources available at the front office.

The decision to admit clients with special needs and specific cultural, ethnic, or religious backgrounds, with which no therapists at the center are familiar, is given special consideration. Such clients are informed of the level of match or mismatch between their stated needs and what is available at the center. Clients may be given a choice to converse with a therapist to discuss what may be needed to meet these special needs. If the client can be accommodated, the admission takes place; if not, a referral is given.

In cases where clients are able to use the services of the center for certain needs, and other services are also appropriate but not available, referrals will be made, and steps will be taken to provide collaborative treatment.

_____ (name of practice) provides interdisciplinary services designed to best accommodate the needs of its clients. Disciplines represented at the center include medical doctors, psychologists, professional counselors, social workers, and marriage and family therapists.

Upon the initial screening, the client is assigned to a therapist who best matches the client's therapeutic needs. Only those clinicians specifically trained and supervised in severe mental illness are assigned to clients with such needs.

The basic components of the program include the use of individual psychotherapy, group therapy, and family-oriented treatment. The use of such modalities as focused process group therapy, group therapy, individual therapy, family therapy, and psychopharmacology will make up the program.

A team approach is employed for the entire scope of client services. The primary therapist conducts the initial intake of the client. Clinic policies and procedures provide guidelines as to determining the extent of services, such as the need for a medication review. In these cases, a clinic referral or an appointment to a clinic psychiatrist is made.

Some clients see more than one therapist within the clinic. The collaboration of services is integrated in the treatment plan. Services such as medication management, individual therapy and group therapy, and relationship therapy necessitates a collaboration between professionals.

Group Therapy

Group therapy meetings will provide confrontation of denial, group identification, expression of feelings, and an attempt for reconstruction. The preferable group size is 6 to 12.

Therapeutic goals include self-understanding, self-acceptance, self-reliance and improved peer interaction. Group therapy will be conducted and facilitated by a professional member of the treatment staff who has been trained in group therapy.

Process groups will discuss educational information that relates to lifestyle changes, and provide a more solid knowledge of basic daily living skills, alternative coping mechanisms, and knowledge of the components of a mentally and physically healthy lifestyle.

Individual Therapy

Individual psychotherapy is conducted to provide individual support, reality orientation, venting of feelings, and insight reconstruction that is necessary for recovery. Control of impulsivity, enhancing the level of ego functioning, and acceptance of responsibility will be emphasized. Within the short-term treatment requirements dictated by current third-party payer requirements, solutions oriented psychotherapy is practiced.

The level and frequency of individual psychotherapy will be assessed on a case-by-case basis. However, weekly individual therapy is an accepted norm.

Family Therapy

Therapeutic interaction may take place by involving an individual family member, and/or through conjunctive therapy, family therapy, or family group. Family involvement in Alanon and Naranon is seen as critical to the recovery process for both the chemically dependent client and their family. When treatment involving the family is ongoing, then aftercare planning for the family will be part of the overall treatment plan.

Family therapy will be conducted by a member of the professional staff, so privileged, and as clinically indicated.

The expected outcome is the stabilization of family relationships in order to support ongoing health. Structured or systematic family oriented therapy will be practiced by those clinicians who are appropriately trained and credentialed.

Aftercare Services

The primary therapist will regularly provide feedback to the referral source regarding admission, continued stay, progress in treatment, and as appropriate, will schedule conferences and aftercare meetings. Clients referred from managed care (or similar) systems will be referred to follow-up treatment approved by or recommended by the referring system. Focus on the importance and necessity of continuing with self-help meeting attendance will be emphasized during treatment, as will other aftercare services.

Issues that were deferred during outpatient treatment will be planned for as part of the aftercare plan. Client involvement in the aftercare plan is fully expected. However, it should be acknowledged that outpatient services are considered the least restrictive level of professional care, and most of our clients are not seen on any other level of professional care once discharged. The exception to this is when a client requires a more intensive level of care and is hospitalized, or referred to residential, partial hospital or day treatment care. Since managed care comprises much of our referral base, the decision of where the client is referred may not be ours or the client's. It is often controlled by the managed care company, and is contractually based.

Services are implemented to support the recovery of the persons served. Treatment plans are implemented to provide a best estimate of the required time frame for necessary treatment. Treatment plans are periodically revised to best refocus the extent, scope, timing, and modality of treatment. Treatment plans are written in a sequential manner, by which progress can be observed and evaluated during the course of treatment.

Appointments are made in a time frame that best meets the client's needs within the parameters of an outpatient clinic.

Psychiatric services are available at the center and through referrals. Related therapeutic, supportive, and psycho-educational services may be referred within the center and to other agencies.

Persons with co-occurring psychiatric disorders or dual diagnosis will receive or be referred to services that address the scope of their needs. The substance abuse program follows the abstinence model.

Following the *DSM* as a guide to defining symptoms of each diagnosis, the confirmation of a mental health diagnosis is based on the impairments experienced by mental health symptoms. Symptom and impairment reduction is the model by which a diagnosis is validated. When concordant symptoms and resultant impairments of a diagnosis are no longer present, it is assumed that treatment (at least under the given diagnosis) is no longer medically necessary.

Restoration of function in a number of areas such as affective, social, occupational, academic, behavioral, and other domains is a primary goal of treatment. Clients seek mental health services due to impairments in functioning in such areas; therefore, restoration of function involves alleviation of such impairments. Treatment plans are written in a manner such that behavioral functioning is measurable, quantifiable, or observable. Outcome measures provide additional evidence of restoration of functioning. Successful treatment is designed to demonstrate these principles.

In order to prevent additional functional impairments, the treatment and aftercare is designed to provide the client the skills necessary to prevent relapse. The comprehensive assessment, and the ongoing information gathering which takes place each session, are intended to identify both areas of strength and weakness. Areas of weakness that are not part of the presenting problem, or occur as the result of environmental changes due to the effects of treatment (e.g., client becomes more assertive, leading to protests from family), are regularly monitored and treated. The course of treatment is considered ever changing, due to the effects of therapy.

SAFETY POLICIES

Safety Procedures

It is important to have written policies and procedures that cover a variety of safety procedures. The goal is to protect both clients and staff. Such P and Ps do not guarantee that an incident will not occur, but may decrease its likelihood through compliance with safety

Sample Safety Practices, Policies, and Procedures

Security is provided for all clients and staff at _____ (name of practice). While _____ (name of practice) cannot guarantee the safety of its clients and staff, every effort is taken to protect and provide for a safe environment.

The parking lot at _____ (name of practice) is lighted, and has automatic timers that come on at dusk and stay on until dawn.

The security of the building is greatly dependent upon the observation of strangers by staff, and by making sure that secure areas are always locked. Security of _____ (name of practice) is the responsibility of all staff.

Whenever possible, the staff should never leave alone and should try to exit the building in groups or pairs. While _____ (name of practice) operations are not located in a high crime area, alertness and common sense can greatly benefit the safety of all parties.

When the facility is not operational, the doors are kept locked and secured. Outside of normal business hours, the main doors to the building are locked and can be opened only by using the coding system specifically designed for _____ (name of practice) employees. This code is given to new staff upon hiring. This code is to remain confidential for safety and security reasons. If it is discovered that the code has been divulged, and the safety and security of the clients and staff has been compromised, the building management will be notified and a new code will be requested.

The facility has operational telephones 24 hours per day, 7 days per week. In the event of a crime or threat to staff or clients, the police can be summoned by dialing 911. Staff who observe a stranger in the facility should try to ascertain who the person is, and what business they have in the facility. If threatened, they should seek other staff members immediately, and should request that the police be summoned. Remember, a calm attitude and an immediate call to the police are the most important actions when confronted with a threatening situation.

An incident report should be filed in the event of a breech of security. These forms are available from the safety officer, or any office or administrative staff member. Completed forms should be turned in immediately to the safety officer.

practices. Keeping a record of safety breeches allows the clinic to observe and correct patterns in problem areas.

Quarterly or monthly practices, such as drills for fires and other disasters and emergencies, help prepare the clinic to deal calmly with the unexpected. Keep a log of each drill. Make notations of the

amount of time each drill takes, with the goal of improving the response time.

Plan for Emergency Services

Wherever groups of people meet, an emergency situation will eventually occur. An emergency services plan defines an emergency and
describes how to handle the situation. Larger clinics typically have
emergency action drills for events such as fires, tornadoes, power
blackouts, bomb threats, or similar emergency events. The plan includes contacts for outside services which may not be available at
the clinic. Typically, each of these events has a separate written
policy.

Bomb Threat Plan

Although the likelihood of a bomb threat may be small, an ounce of
prevention certainly could be a lifesaver should the event occur. Although smaller clinics likely will not have personnel with assigned
titles such as a safety officer, there should be an established chain
of command in a clinic for when key personnel are not present. That
is, for various reasons and purposes, there should always be someone in a key decision making role.

Fire Extinguisher and Warning Procedures

Clinic personnel will be trained in the use of fire extinguishers. A
brief training in a staff meeting that goes over the policies, procedures and locations of fire extinguishers could make a major different in the event of a fire.

Sample Plan for Emergency Services

As part of its program to provide a safe and healthy environment, at _____ (name of practice) has developed this *Plan for Emergency Services* to assure that patients and staff handle emergency conditions appropriately.

The executive director or a designee is responsible for developing safety related policies and procedures throughout the facility. These policies and procedures include those related to emergencies. During orientation, each staff member is instructed on how to appropriately handle incidents, accidents, and natural disasters, including the emergency measures to be taken. The executive committee regularly evaluates the implementation of these measures. A reportable incident is defined as any unusual occurrence outside the normal activities of the facility. Incidents should be reported whether they occur within the facility, the parking lot, or other parts of the building.

The following are considered to be medical emergencies:

- Injuries resulting from accidents or natural disasters within the facility.

- Symptoms of life threatening illness, such as hemorrhaging, breathing difficulty, severe pain, seizures, or fainting.

- Physical complaints that might be indicative of a life threatening condition, such as dizziness, irregular heartbeat combined with loss of color, or high fever combined with behavioral change.

- Spontaneous labor in a pregnant female.

- Ingestion of alcohol or drugs resulting in inability to function safely within the clinical environment.

- Any other incident or physical symptom considered by the staff to put a patient or a staff member at risk. The professional judgment of the staff is respected, since it is better to ask for services that are not needed than to need services that are not requested.

The following are considered to be mental emergencies:

- Disorientation to time, place, or person.

- Bizarre behavior indicating loss of touch with reality.

- Threat of harm to self or others.

- Actual violence to self or others.

- Any other incident or mental symptom considered by the staff to put a patient or a staff member at risk.

Since the facility is not equipped to handle these physical and mental emergencies, _____ (name of practice) has established referral agreements with other facilities.

Medical emergencies are handled by the following facilities:

(Names and phone numbers)

Mental emergencies are handled by the following facilities:

(Names and phone numbers)

Emergencies requiring detoxification services are handled by the following facilities:

(Names and phone numbers)

Further information on these facilities is kept readily available in the *Referral Resource Manual* kept at the front desk.

When such emergencies arise, the executive director evaluates the situation, administers appropriate attention, supervises transfer, and sees that the appropriate information is transmitted. In the absence of the executive director, the ranking staff member is in charge.

An office support staff member calls for ambulance or police support, notifies the emergency facility of the impending transport, and notifies the client's family of the circumstances. The executive director or ranking staff member assigns the responsibility to someone else if necessary. Ambulance service is (name, address, phone). When written records are requested by the emergency facility, all rules of confidentiality are observed. An incident report will be filled out by the staff member who handled the emergency, and filed in the *Incident Report Log* within 24 hours.

Sample Bomb Threat Plan

Notification and Warning

1. Most bomb threats are made by telephone or by mail. The first staff person notified of the threat of a bomb should remain calm and try to gather as much information as possible. That person should immediately notify another staff member to notify the police and building management, as well as the safety officer. If the threat is made verbally, the staff person receiving the call should attempt to log any identifying information such as the gender and ethnicity of the caller, distinguishing background noises, dialect, distinctive phrases, and so on. The staff member should remember, to the best of their ability, the exact verbiage used by the caller. If possible, the staff member should write down what is said while the caller is speaking. The staff person should obtain and fill out a *Bomb Threat Documentation* form.

2. All staff at _____ (name of practice) are trained on procedures regarding bomb threats and evacuation. The primary responsibility for all staff is to warn clients and evacuate as soon as possible. Except for the items listed above, the evacuation plan used is the same as that used for fire evacuations.

General Responses

1. If a bomb threat is reported, the receiving staff member should notify the safety officer immediately. If the safety officer is not on-site at this time, the highest-ranking administrator present at the time of the threat should be notified. The safety officer, or a designee, will notify all staff to evacuate the building immediately.

2. Staff should escort their clients, leave their office doors open, and evacuate the building by following their emergency evacuation maps to the outside of the building. The office personnel will be responsible for attending to all clients and family members in the lobby, and escorting them out of the building. All staff should report to the center of the rear of the parking lot.

3. One office staff person shall be responsible for removal of the office scheduling books. These books will be utilized to make sure all persons are accounted for. This staff member should also make sure the *Bomb Threat Documentation* form is taken outside during the evacuation.

4. The safety officer, or a designee, will make a final run through of the entire suite, verifying that all offices and work areas have been evacuated.

5. Clinicians will account for their clients and family members in the sheltered area, and report this information to the safety officer, or a designee.

6. The safety officer, or a designee, shall take roll of all clients and staff once outside to ensure that all occupants are evacuated. Any missing person will be reported to the fire department immediately upon arrival. The building management shall notify other residents of the building.

Remember, the primary responsibility is to warn the occupants of the building, to evacuate immediately, and to notify the police department and building management of the bomb threat.

Evacuation drills shall be held quarterly, and the safety officer shall record the time needed to evacuate the building. The facility shall be evacuated in 3 minutes or less. The administrator shall evaluate the results of the drills, and shall report the results in the quarterly report.

Sample Fire Disaster Plan

Notification and Warning

1. The first staff person to notice the fire should immediately notify another staff person to call 911 to report the fire and its location to the fire department.

2. The staff persons observing the fire will pull the fire alarm, notifying all staff to evacuate the building. Fire alarms are located next to the stairwells leading to the main floor.

3. If the fire is small and can be extinguished easily, it should be put out by a staff person using a fire extinguisher. All staff at _____ (name of practice) are trained in the use of fire extinguishers. The primary responsibility of all staff is to warn and evacuate as soon as possible.

4. _____ (name of practice) uses the acronym R.A.C.E. (Rescue, Alert, Contain, Evacuate) to outline fire emergency procedures.

General Response

1. If a fire is reported, staff should take the appropriate precautions to keep their clients safe from harm. Staff members should always feel doors to determine if they are hot and possibly hiding a fire. Do not open a door if it is hot, a hidden fire can cause a back draft. Most suites have two separate means of egress. The staff member should determine which means would be the most safe.

2. If trapped by a fire, remain calm and notify someone of your location and condition. Attempt to slow smoke inhalation by blocking off gaps at the bottom of the door with clothing or other materials that can slow smoke coming into the room.

3. Once it is deemed safe to exit the office, staff should escort their clients, leave their office doors open, and evacuate the building by following their emergency evacuation maps to the outside of the building. Office personnel will be responsible for attending to all clients and family members in the lobby, and escorting them out of the building. All staff should escort their clients and report to the center of the rear of the parking lot.

4. One office staff person shall be responsible for removal of the office scheduling books. These books will be utilized to make sure all persons are accounted for.

5. The safety officer, or a designee, will make a final run-through of the entire suite, verifying that all offices and work areas have been evacuated, and closing all doors and windows. This will ensure that there will be no drafts to fan the fire or allow the smoke to circulate.

6. Clinicians will account for their clients and family members in the sheltered area, and report this information to the safety officer, or a designee.

7. The safety officer, or a designee, shall take roll of all clients and staff once outside to ensure that all occupants are evacuated. Any missing person will be reported immediately upon arrival of the fire department. Other residents of the building shall be notified of the fire by the fire alarm, and/or the ranking administrator, if necessary.

8. The ranking administrator, or a designee, shall direct the fire department to the location of the fire.

Remember, the primary responsibility is to warn the occupants of the building, to evacuate immediately and to notify the fire department of the fire and its location.

Fire drills shall be held quarterly. The safety officer shall record the time taken to evacuate the building. The facility shall be evacuated in 3 minutes or less.

The administrator shall evaluate the results of the fire drills, and shall report the results in the minutes of the quarterly report.

Sample Fire Extinguisher and Warning Procedures

Fire extinguishers are kept readily available in all areas of _____ (name of practice). There are _____ (number of extinguishers) extinguishers located in the suite. The locations are listed below:

(List locations of fire extinguishers)

Note: Also provide the specific locations of fire extinguishers in the building on a diagram of the building.

The facility safety officer, as part of the monthly safety inspection, checks the extinguishers. The extinguisher company that services and replaces the fire extinguishers also checks extinguishers annually. The monthly safety and cleanliness inspections document the condition of the extinguishers and this information is reported to the administrator. The annual report by the extinguisher company will be included with the safety checklist. In the event that an extinguisher is found to be inactive, or less than safe, the ranking administrator will be notified immediately. If an extinguisher is discharged, the extinguisher company should replace it immediately. The safety office shall notify the company of the need for a new extinguisher.

If a fire is noticed, the staff person should decide if the fire is able to be extinguished by a fire extinguisher. The most important thing is the safety of clients and staff. If there is any question, the staff person witnessing the fire should contact another staff person and have him or her inform administration and call 911. If the fire is small and can be extinguished easily, it should be put out by a staff person trained on fire extinguisher use. Remember, the primary responsibility for all staff is to extinguish, warn, and evacuate when appropriate, as soon as possible.

Fire Disaster and Fire Extinguisher Acronyms

Each staff person will be trained on the use of fire extinguishers. The PASS acronym is utilized in the training process.

P **P**ull the pin

A **A**im the nozzle at the base of the flame

S **S**queeze the handle to expel the extinguisher's contents

S **S**weep the base of the flame

The RACE acronym is also referred to in a _____ (name of practice) fire disaster.

R Rescue

A Alarm

C Contain

E Evacuate

Severe Weather Procedures

During times of severe weather prompt decisions are necessary to ensure the safety of clients and staff. Procedures must be in place to deal with both staff and clients at the facility, and those who have appointments. Always have regular and alternate phone numbers, or other means of contacting all clients and staff.

Tornado Procedures

Tornadoes are more serious than severe weather, and proper procedures must be followed strictly. In case of a tornado there must be a designated shelter area for staff and clients. It is suggested that therapists remain with their clients, and staff be accountable for those in the waiting room. As in fire drills, education about tornado procedures can eliminate much confusion when the actual event occurs.

SUMMARY

Written policies and procedures, in themselves, can seem like tedious tasks placed upon a clinic and its employees. However, when emergencies or uncertainties arise, they can be the only thread that keeps everyone together during the crisis. Very specific P and Ps are required by accrediting agencies and many of them, just as a business plan, are typically required when applying for a business loan.

Sample Severe Weather Procedures Policy

Notification and Warning

1. Notification of a severe weather watch or warning is received by commercial radio, television and/or by client or staff member with confirmation.

2. In the event that a weather emergency is declared during working hours, the safety officer, or a designee, will communicate this information to the staff by way of the telephone, public address system, or a door-to-door announcement. In the event that an emergency is declared during hours in which the facility is not open, the CEO* will either (a) contact local radio stations informing them that the facility will not open, and/or (b) contact the safety officer to have him or her notify all personnel by telephone.

General Response

1. When a severe weather watch is issued, the safety officer will monitor weather conditions, or designate another employee to do so.

2. If a severe weather warning is issued, personnel may be released early, as deemed appropriate. Onsite operations may be minimized or curtailed, as necessary.

3. Personnel released early will be recalled by telephone when conditions permit.

4. If a decision is made to close the facility, the safety officer, designee, and/or a therapist is responsible for contacting the clients so they may be informed that sessions will not be held.

5. In the event that sessions are in progress, and a decision is made to close the facility, the staff should ensure that all clients have transportation home. If not, arrangements should be coordinated with family members or the local authorities (i.e., police and fire departments, and the county sheriff department).

6. In the event of danger from lightning, the safety officer is responsible for ensuring that the computer system and all units are shut down.

*In the absence of the CEO, the safety officer, administrator, administrative coordinator, or a designee, shall function in his or her stead.

Sample Tornado Procedures

Notification and Warning

1. Notification of a tornado warning is received by local sirens, and/or commercial radio, television, or a confirmed report by a client or staff member.

2. When a tornado watch is issued, or when severe or threatening weather conditions exist, the safety officer may designate personnel to monitor the weather for an upgrade to a tornado warning. If the safety officer is not in the office, another administrative person or designee will take on those responsibilities.

3. Personnel sighting a funnel cloud should immediately report it to the police department by calling 911. The funnel cloud sighting should then be immediately reported to the safety officer or another administrative person for notification of all staff and clients.

4. The safety officer, or designee, should announce the warning through the telephone public address system or go door-to-door and announce the immediate evacuation of the suite per the procedure listed below.

General Response

1. When a tornado watch is issued, the safety officer, or a designee, will monitor weather conditions, or designate a staff member as weather monitor.

2. The safety officer, or a designee, will alert all staff of a tornado warning. Each staff member is responsible for the care and safety of their client. The office staff personnel will care for family members and clients located in the waiting room at the time of the warning.

3. If a tornado warning is issued, staff and clients should seek protective shelter by leaving their doors open and following their emergency evacuation route to (list where to go in your building). All persons should stay away from all glass areas once in the first floor hallway. Emergency doors shall be closed to protect all persons from possible flying glass from the lobby windows should a tornado, high winds, or flying debris damage the building.

4. One office staff person shall be responsible for removal of the office scheduling books. These books will be utilized to make sure all persons are accounted for.

5. The safety officer, or a designee, will make a final run-through of the entire suite, verifying that all offices and work areas are vacant, and close all doors.

> 6. Clinicians will account for their clients and family members in the sheltered area, and report this information to the safety officer, or a designee.
>
> 7. When the tornado warning is cancelled or downgraded, the safety officer, or a designee, will determine if continued weather monitoring is advisable, and take the appropriate steps.
>
> 8. Personnel will remain in the sheltered area until the all clear notice is given. Again, the sheltered area is on the main floor, in the central hallway, away from all glass areas. Once notice is given, therapists should escort their clients back to their offices.

P and Ps allow the clinic to run smoothly, and for clinic actions to be uniform and fair to both employees and clients. Clients who receive services from different therapists can be assured that policies such as admission requirements, billing procedures, the fee schedule, and any other aspects of clinic business are not unfair. In addition, with adequate P and Ps staff know their job requirements and parameters.

Outside agencies, such as accrediting agencies and third-party payers, carefully scrutinize the clinic's P and Ps to evaluate the quality of services and business practices.

Within the clinic, when employees are trained in and required to read the P and Ps, they provide the clinic with a level of protection by adherence to solid ethical, therapeutic, and business practices.

TEST YOUR KNOWLEDGE

1. Policies and procedures are important because, when followed, they
   - (a) keep administrators busy.
   - (b) can prevent confusion in uncertain situations.
   - (c) provide evidence that a clinic can follow the rules.
   - (d) reduce the need for management.

2. Besides helping in clinic operations, policies and procedures may be needed to

    (a) secure a loan.

    (b) obtain insurance payments.

    (c) receive health insurance for employees of a clinic.

    (d) receive county contracts.

3. A clinic without policies and procedures may be liable for a client's injury

    (a) when the lack of procedures led to or exacerbated the injury or prevented prompt treatment.

    (b) outside of the clinic, if the client is on the way home from a session when injured.

    (c) if employees are not trained in first-aid.

    (d) in none of these cases.

4. A client denied admission to a clinic is more likely to understand the reason for the denial and not view it as discriminatory when

    (a) there are no other clients at the clinic with similar concerns.

    (b) there is a referral given to another clinic.

    (c) specific admission criteria are published.

    (d) the client has a high level of insight.

Answers: 1. b; 2. d; 3. a; 4. c

10

Documentation Procedures

This book contains a chapter about documentation procedures because evaluating these procedures is one of the primary duties of a clinic director or clinical manager. This duty includes training clinicians and monitoring their work. This chapter provides examples and training in the area of documentation required by third-party payers, licensure agencies, and accrediting organizations.

THE IMPORTANCE OF DOCUMENTATION

If you have ever been subject to an insurance company audit you clearly know the importance of documentation. Although most audits seem to take place in larger clinics, small clinics and one-person private practices are not immune.

Accountability is the keystone of ethical and professional practice. In the field of mental health, typically only the therapist and client truly know what takes place in a session. For those with a high degree of professionalism, it is assumed that the treatment they provide is helpful, current, and efficacious. However, it cannot be assumed that every therapist practices at this level. As in other professional fields, there must be evidence or documentation that the services provided are helpful. In addition, when third-party payment is involved, services must also be medically necessary. That is, without such services the client is likely to decline, or not improve, in a reasonable amount of time.

What Takes Place in an Audit?

Typically, one or more auditors contact the clinic and announce an upcoming audit, which will take place in a relatively brief period of time. Sometimes they ask to review specific charts, while at other times they review charts at random. The auditors are given full access to the charts of clients whose services were paid for by the company the auditors represent. Your contract with the third-party payer covers such provisions.

The charts selected for review are carefully scrutinized in several areas to determine the necessity and appropriateness of services. This is determined solely by documentation. Thus, even if services were medically necessary, and the quality of services was superior and resulted in successful mental health functioning, if the course of treatment is not adequately documented, you may be required to pay back all of the funds paid for the services.

Auditors review documentation for the intake, diagnosis, treatment plan, progress notes, length of services, and how these elements interrelate. For example, the treatment plan must be concordant with the intake material. The progress notes must consistently follow the treatment plan and regularly validate the need for services. When there are discrepancies, such as a progress note that is unclear, vague, does not follow the treatment plan, or does not demonstrate the need for services, it is possible that the third party will request that payment is returned for all or some of the services provided to the client. If the intake does not clearly document the need for services, all money received may have to be paid back.

With adequate documentation of services, an objective third party (e.g., supervisor, payer, accrediting association, state board) is able to review the records (documentation) to help determine if the course of services is appropriate, on target, and timely. Without mandates for adequate documentation, the costs of mental health insurance can be affected, due to some therapists providing an excessive number of sessions when such services may not have been necessary.

Poor documentation is very problematic because it produces little or scattered evidence in areas such as the diagnosis, symptoms, impairments, treatment, strengths, weaknesses, effect of services, and so on. Without clear documentation, clinical supervision becomes much more difficult. When third parties conduct an audit of records, they do not contact clients or discuss cases with thera-pists; they only review the records.

Documentation may have little to do with the quality of the counseling taking place, but without good documentation it is pos-sible that a client in need of additional services could be denied those services. The denial would not necessarily stem from an un-caring auditor or case manager, but from the therapist's lack of ev-idence that additional services are needed.

This chapter provides training in several areas of documenta-tion, covering all areas of treatment from the initial intake to the discharge. It is presented in an atheoretical manner, from the view-point of no particular school of thought. Documentation is presented in terms or measurable behaviors, but has nothing to do with behav-ioral therapy. Those who review documentation desire an empirical model, or the medical model, because progress can be measured, rather than implied. Anyone involved in clinic direction/manage-ment must be well versed in documentation procedures.

BASIC CONCEPTS OF DOCUMENTATION

The following section is provided for case managers, clinical super-visors, and others who review client files. It includes common third-party requirements, with examples of acceptable and unacceptable documentation.

Document with Empirical Evidence

Documentation is about empirical evidence. Opinions and hunches may be important in therapy, but do not state them as facts or evi-dence in documentation. Evidence is written in a manner that clearly defines the problem area.

Poor example of documenting that a client is depressed:
Victoria K. is depressed most of the time and meets the crite-ria for Major Depressive Disorder.

Problem: It does not validate the *DSM* criteria for a depressive episode, and does not describe impairments that validate her need for treatment.

Good example of documenting that a client is depressed:

Victoria K. states that she has felt depressed for the past 3 months since she broke up with her fiancé. Since that time she has missed work about 50 percent of the time, and has not spent any time with friends or family, as she had in the past on a regular basis. She states that she is depressed most of the time, has few pleasures in life, has a very low appetite (leading to losing 35 pounds), and has regular thoughts of death. Typically, it takes her over 2 hours to fall asleep, and she wakes at least hourly. She further notes, "I have no motivation to do anything. I just exist. Who cares anymore? Can you help me?"

Why is it better?

Although this passage may take more time to write than the first example, it provides a much clearer picture of the client's symptoms and impairments. Specific examples are given along with client quotes. The examples are empirical because we know how much work she is missing, the amount of time she spends with friends, how much weight she has lost, her amount of sleep, and other, less empirical, descriptions. If someone was reviewing her case, this statement would provide ample evidence that she meets the *DSM* requirements for Major Depressive Disorder, and needs treatment.

Use of the OFAID Procedure

The OFAID procedure is a method of documenting mental health symptoms, and compares levels of impairment throughout treatment. It provides a baseline and current levels of a number of areas of functioning. The acronym OFAID stands for:

Onset

When did the current mental health concerns begin? Many diagnoses have a time period placed on the onset of symptoms.

Example: Liz began exhibiting temper tantrums in the last year, shortly after her father left home.

Frequency

How frequently does it take place?

  Example: Liz throws tantrums at least five times per day.

Antecedents

What triggers it to happen?

  Example: Liz throws tantrums almost every time she does not get her way.

Intensity

How severe are the symptoms/impairments?

  Example: Liz's mother rates her severity of tantrums as a 9 out of 10 based on associated behaviors of head banging, property destruction, and assaults on family members.

Duration

How long do the symptoms last?

  Example: Liz's tantrums typically last 30 to 60 minutes.

Good and bad examples of OFAID procedure:
Whenever it is possible, incorporate the OFAID variables in documentation. They provide an excellent means of validating a diagnosis, measuring and comparing levels of progress, and determining when to terminate treatment.

Poor example:
  Cynthia B. is seeking an evaluation because she is anxious and has Panic Attacks.
  Problem: We do not know the level or reasons for her symptoms. We have no idea whether her Panic Attacks are minor or debilitating. Without this information we have no basis to determine the level of treatment necessary, or if the level of symptoms and impairments are at a diagnosable level.

Good example:
  Cynthia B. began having Panic Attacks 2 months ago (onset) since she was humiliated at her high school reunion. She experi-

ences panic symptoms about twice per day (frequency), whenever she tries to go outside or anticipates going outside (antecedents). She rates their severity as a 90 on a 100-point scale, noting that she often feels like passing out, her chest hurts, she has trouble breathing, she has palpitations, she trembles, and must flee the situation or symptoms increase (*DSM* symptoms criteria). Most of these symptoms last about 15 to 20 minutes (duration). She is now avoiding friends and has not returned to work (impairments).

Why is it better?

The OFAID procedure provides a clearer overview of the course of her Panic Attacks. The information can be used in her treatment planning to monitor and validate therapeutic progress. For example, if Panic Attacks initially lasted an average of 20 minutes, but after a number of therapy sessions they decreased to an average of 10 minutes, there appears to be some progress. In addition, we can also monitor the frequency and intensity of symptoms and impairments. An example of monitoring frequency of impairments, in this example, is "Over the past month she has missed work 60 percent of the time, but after 2 months of treatment she is missing work no more than 15 percent of the time due to Panic Attacks." In addition, the passage validates the *DSM* criteria of symptoms and impairments.

Provide Treatment That Is Concordant with Acceptable Standards

The field of mental health treatment is backed by a myriad of research. Numerous texts describe which therapies tend to be most helpful for various diagnoses and problem areas. It is not uncommon for a contract with a third-party payer to state that treatment methods must be those that have been proven to be effective. There is often a clause that experimental therapies are not covered. If you provide a type of treatment that is either new, experimental, or nontraditional, and third-party payment is involved, I suggest that you first check with a case manager for approval to conduct the type of treatment in question.

Five Means of Obtaining Clinical Data for Documentation

When documenting mental health information there are several possible sources of data. Relying on only one source may be risky. For example, if a client is in denial, has poor insight, or is malingering, the information received will be flawed, leading to incorrect or incomplete conclusions. As additional sources of information increase, the level of confidence in your results increases. Data for documentation can come from at least five possible sources. If you are in a position in which you supervise therapists, encourage them to collect data from multiple sources.

1. *Clinical Observations:* Behaviors observed by the therapist

    Example: "The client appeared to be anxious and depressed."

2. *Client Statements:* Specific statements made by the client

    Example: The client stated, "I have no reason to live."

3. *Testing:* Objective, standardized test results

    Example: "MMPI-2 results indicated at Scale 2 (Depression) *t*-score of 110, suggesting significant concerns in depression at this time."

4. *Previous Records:* Past psychological records

    Example: "Records from Bayo Clinic on Jan. 2, 2007, indicated a diagnosis of Major Depressive Disorder, moderate, without psychotic features."

5. *Collateral Information:* Information received from other information

    Example: "The client's spouse states that the client appears depressed most of the time, misses work most days, seldom eats, and avoids most people."

THIRD-PARTY AND ACCREDITATION REQUIREMENTS

A book of this size certainly cannot go over every requirement for documentation, but the major points will be covered. The following documentation requirements are taken from various auditor's checklists. The same information is very helpful for those providing clinical supervision.

The Initial Interview: Validating Symptoms, Impairments, and the Diagnosis

The initial interview is extremely important in documentation. It sets the stage for the treatment plan and the course of therapy. Therefore, the first session is more about collecting information than counseling. The primary goals of the initial interview are to clearly define the client's concerns, and formulate a diagnosis and treatment plan.

The purpose of this text is not how to conduct a diagnostic interview, but rather, it teaches what to document. The *DSM* clearly defines a mental health diagnosis in terms of symptoms and impairments. Each diagnosis lists a number of symptoms that define that diagnosis.

Validating Symptoms

Diagnoses are further broken down by essential and associated symptoms. Most diagnoses list at least one essential symptom that must be present, and other symptoms, of which a certain number must be present in order to give the diagnosis. Thus, whenever reviewing a file be sure that the documentation of the diagnosis fits the *DSM* criteria for symptoms. Consider the following two examples.

Poor example of validating symptoms of a diagnosis:
"The client is depressed. Symptoms are most concordant with a diagnosis of Major Depressive Disorder."
Problem: There is not a validation of symptoms according to the *DSM* criteria.

Good example of validating symptoms of a diagnosis:
"The client states that he has been depressed most of the time for the past 3 months. He states that he has few or no pleasures in

Provide Therapists With the Necessary Tools to Document

As a clinical supervisor, be sure that the therapists you supervise have adequate forms to record information, and ample time to validate *DSM* diagnostic information. Without such a system, documentation can become quite difficult. Provide them with training so that they are thoroughly familiar with the *DSM* and the forms used in your clinic. Make them aware of the requirements of each third-party payer and accrediting agencies, if your clinic is accredited. Information is power.

his life, has lost 25 pounds, has a significantly decreased appetite, avoids other people, has increasing thoughts of death, and cannot sleep more than an hour at a time. Symptoms are concordant with a diagnosis of Major Depressive Disorder."

Why is it better?

The *DSM-IV-TR* lists the essential features of a Major Depressive Episode as having at least five of nine listed symptoms for at least a 2-week period, of which either being depressed most of the time, or lack of pleasure must be one of the symptoms. As in some other diagnoses, time factors and symptoms are listed. Thus, in any diagnostic interview the clinician must be aware of the essential and associated symptoms in order to rule in or rule out the diagnostic possibilities.

When making statements in a diagnostic report be sure that the intake material validates the previous statements. That is, simply stating that the client has these symptoms is not enough. It should be validated by material such as client checklists, testing, interview sheets, or other material demonstrating that the client endorsed such symptoms. An auditor should be able to locate in the files that such symptoms have been endorsed.

Validating Impairments

DSM symptoms define a diagnosis, but are not sufficient to make a diagnosis. The introduction of the *DSM* defines a mental disorder as the existence of symptoms, as described previously in this chapter, but there must also be functional impairments, a significant risk, or loss of freedom as a result of the disorder. Thus, documentation must also include a description of symptoms and impairments.

Impairments resultant from a mental health disorder may be experienced in a number of ways, such as socially, occupationally, academically, in terms of psychological stress, or other areas significantly interfering with the client's functioning. As with symptoms, impairments must be validated to further confirm the diagnosis. When possible, document impairments in a format such as the previously mentioned OFAID procedure. This information will be very helpful in planning treatment.

Poor example of documenting impairments:
"Devin L. is having difficulty in school."
Problem:
When validating impairments there should be examples of how they are the result of a mental health disorder, and should clearly describe an impaired condition at a level lower than premorbid functioning.

Good example of documenting impairments:
"Since breaking up with her fiancé 2 months ago, Devin L.'s grades have dropped from an A– average, to no grade higher than a D. Her attendance has changed from perfect attendance to missing 50 percent of her college classes. She received a letter from the academic dean that she is now on academic probation, and is in danger of failing all of her classes."
Why is it better?
Documentation of impairments provides ample evidence of the need for mental health treatment. The main documentation issue is to link the impairments to the symptoms. The previous example is more complete when both symptoms and resultant impairments are documented, as follows:
"Devin L. states that she has Panic Attacks at least six times per week, which last about 20 to 30 minutes, primarily when she leaves the house. She endorses the following symptoms: palpitations, trembling, shortness of breath, chest pain, fear of dying, and chills. She rates the Subjective Units of Distress (SUD) of her Panic Attacks at 90 out of 100 possible units of distress. Symptoms have taken place since

breaking up with her fiancé 2 months ago. Her grades have dropped from an A– average, to no grade higher than a D. Her attendance has changed from perfect attendance to missing 50 percent of her college classes. She received a letter from the academic dean that she is now on academic probation, and is in danger of failing all of her courses."

TREATMENT PLANS

The treatment plan is perhaps the foremost document in clients' files. It can be compared to a contract or a blueprint, describing the client's problem areas and how they will be treated. It includes measurable means to evaluate client progress and setbacks. Estimated time frames for treatment, along with treatment modalities and referrals, are included.

The job of an auditor or clinical supervisor is to review the intake material, treatment plans, and progress notes to evaluate how well these coordinate with each other and substantiate the medical necessity of services. The material listed in the treatment plan must follow the intake information, and the progress notes must follow the treatment plan.

Treatment plans are intended to be written in an objective, measurable manner. Just as a builder follows a blueprint, therapy follows a treatment plan. In either case revisions can be made, but each involves an understanding and an agreement between the therapist and client. The treatment plan is always written collaboratively, with specific goals and objectives designed to be met in the course of mental health treatment. The information written in a treatment plan is solely based on information received in the intake and subsequent sessions. The plan focuses on listing various impairments, setting attainable goals and objectives to increase the client's functioning, and the treatment that will be conducted to attain these goals. Additionally, a treatment plan includes target dates for each objective. The previous client information can now be transformed into a three-column treatment plan covering (1) problem areas, (2) goals and objectives, and (3) treatment strategies.

Although there is not a standard format for a treatment plan, a three-column treatment plan is common.

Three-Column Treatment Plan Format

Column One: Problem Areas

The first column of a treatment plan briefly describes the problem areas that will be treated. Typically, they are written as the impairments that the client describes that brought him or her to therapy. They are usually not *DSM* symptoms unless the symptom is measurable. For example, a symptom of weight loss or gain is easily measurable, but a symptom of low motivation is difficult to measure.

In the previous example, possible problem areas include experiencing Panic Attacks, missing school, and declining school grades, in which the impairments are physical and emotional from the attacks, plus academic due to being at risk of failing courses.

They should correspond to the client's presenting problem, intake material, and diagnosis. Since they follow a diagnosis they should be problem areas that, if not treated, will cause the client to decline in functioning or remain in an impaired condition (medical necessity). They should be written in a manner so that they can be measured and evaluated throughout treatment. Good and poor examples are listed in the following.

Problem Areas	**Why is it a poor or good example?**
Poor example #1 Missing work	*Why is it poor?* Everyone misses some work at times. We do not know the extent of the problem and do not know if it is due to a mental health problem.
Good example #1 Absent from work 50% of the time due to low motivation, suicidal ideations, and crying spells. In danger of losing job if attendance does not reach 95% by June 1.	*Why is it good?* The problem area provides an objective baseline (50%) of the frequency of absences from work. It further links the absences to mental health symptoms. Plus, we validate *DSM-IV* criteria by listing the area of impairment (occupational). It further allows a time period by which the objectives can be incorporated into the treatment plan.

Poor example #2
Low grades in school

Why is it poor?
Not everyone has high grades in school. Some people, for a variety of reasons, don't perform well in school. Low grades, in themselves, do not necessarily suggest a mental health disorder, or a learning disability.

Good example #2
Grades in school have declined from an A– to a D– average since breaking up with her fiancé last term.

Why is it good?
We know the client's previous grade level of an A–; thus, we have a specific goal to reach from the current D– level. We further know the antecedent from which the grades have dropped. It suggests that an emotional impairment has led to an academic impairment. It allows us to set up specific treatment strategies to deal with both academic and emotional issues.

Poor example #3
Panic Attacks

Why is it poor?
We do not know the intensity of the Panic Attacks, nor do we know the resultant impairments. That is, the problem area is much too vague.

Good example #3
Panic Attacks; 3 per day, lasting 30 minutes, resulting in leaving the house no more than once per week. Previously no Panic Attacks, or any difficulties leaving the house or going out with friends.

Why is it good?
We know the frequency and duration of the Panic Attacks. Plus, we know that there are social impairments through the client's changes in socialization and going out of the house.

Column Two: Goals / Objectives

Goals are the desired end result of treatment for each problem area. It is difficult to measure goals. Objectives are the incremental, objective, and measurable steps to meet these goals. The written objectives are behaviors that have become impaired due to the mental health issues. Typically, a problem area has one written goal, and about three objectives to reach that goal in the treatment plan. Objectives are written in such a manner that progress can be demonstrated as outcomes. For example, if someone is so depressed that he is avoiding all of his friends, who he used to see at least three times per week, the objectives should lead incrementally back to being with friends three times per week.

Since objectives are measurable and observable, it is helpful to provide a baseline by which progress may be measured. For example, if a client previously attended work 5 days per week, but due to a mental illness she or he attends work an average of 2.5 days per week, the initial objective may be to increase attendance to a minimum of 4 days per week by a certain target date. The eventual goal will be met when the client is no longer impaired in that area, as evidenced by returning to a premorbid functioning level of consistently working 5 days per week.

Each objective is given a target date. Thus, for example, if this person begins therapy on May 1, there could be an objective to meet with friends at least once per week by May 22, with additional increases as therapy progresses. At any time during treatment the client's progress and setbacks can be monitored to evaluate and make changes in treatment as needed. The following examples of goals and objectives are given using the previously identified problem areas.

Problem Areas	**Goals/Objectives**
Example #1	*Goal #1: Alleviate depressed mood*
Depressed mood resulting in absence from work 50% of the time due to low motivation, suicidal ideations, and daily crying spells. In danger of losing job if attendance does not reach 95% by July 1.	Objectives: 1a—Attendance at work to at least 80% by June 22. 1b—Decrease frequency of crying spells to one or less per week by June 29. 1c—Decrease subjective level of suicidality from current SUD of 90 to 65 or less by June 29.

Example #2
Grades in school have declined from an A– to a D– average since breaking up with her fiancé last term. Previously studied at least 1 hour per day; currently studies no more than 10 minutes per day.

Goal #2: Increase grades to previous level
Objectives:
2a—Increase study time to at least 30 minutes/day by June 20.
2b—Increase average school grades to at least C+ by June 22.

Example #3
Panic Attacks; 3 per day, lasting 30 minutes, resulting in leaving the house no more than once per week. SUD level = 90 Previously no Panic Attacks or any difficulties leaving the house or going out with friends.

Goal #3: Alleviate Panic Attacks
Objectives:
3a—Decrease number of Panic Attacks to 2 or less per day by June 15.
3b—Decrease duration of Panic Attacks to 10 minutes or less by June 15.
3c—Decrease intensity of Panic Attacks to under SUD level of 60 by June 15.

Column Three: Treatment Strategies

The third column is intended to describe the mental health treatment that will be provided for each problem area. The treatment should coincide with current, acceptable means of treating clients, and be within the competencies of the assigned therapist. It should also include other treatment information such as the type of therapy (e.g., individual, group, family), homework assignments, referrals, and other treatment conducted outside of the session. It is common to write the estimated number of sessions for each type of therapy either in this column or in a separate place in the treatment plan.

Using the OFAID procedure with the previous example of Devin L.:

Interview Statements	OFAID
Devin L. states that she has Panic Attacks at least 6 times per week	**F**requency—Panic Attacks at least 6 times per week
That last about 20–30 min	**D**uration—20–30 min
Primarily when she leaves the house	**A**ntecedents—when leaving the house
Since she broke up with her fiancé 2 months ago	**O**nset—2 months ago
SUD of 90	**I**ntensity—90 out of 100
Her grades have dropped from A–s to Ds	**I**ntensity—degree of grade changes of A–s to Ds
Her attendance has changed from perfect attendance to missing 50%	**F**requency—100% to 50%

Poor example of a treatment plan incorporating the previous information:

Problem Areas	Goals/Objectives	Treatment Strategies
1. Panic Attacks	Eliminate Panic Attacks	Individual therapy
2. Declining grades	Increase grades	Individual therapy
3. Declining attendance	Increase attendance	Individual therapy

Problems with a Vague Treatment Plan

This treatment plan is extremely vague. The reader has no idea of the severity or nature of the client's impairments. For example, it is not known how frequent or severe the panic attacks are. The notations of declining grades and attendance do not provide a clue as to the severity of the decline. The goals of increasing grades and attendance provide little indication if they need to be increased significantly, or to a minor amount. The reader does not know the level of dysfunction or impairment. In addition, the type of therapy and the amount of time estimated are not indicated. There is no indication of medical necessity. Overall, the treatment plan does not provide enough evidence that treatment is necessary.

Good example of a treatment plan incorporating the previous information:

Estimated number of sessions: Individual therapy, 12 sessions

Problem Areas	Goals/Objectives	Treatment Strategies
1. Panic Attacks resulting in academic, physical, and affective impairment	(a) Decrease frequency of Panic Attacks to ≤ 3 per week by July 19 Baseline 6 per week (b) Decrease duration of Panic Attacks to ≤ 10 min by July 19 Baseline: 20–30 min each (c) Decrease intensity of Panic Attacks to SUD ≤ 60 by July 19 Baseline: SUD = 90	Cognitive behavioral Relaxation Analyzing negative thoughts
2. Declining school performance, resulting in potentially failing grades	(a) Increase attendance to ≥ 90% by July 14 Baseline: 50% (b) Increase school grades to ≥ C+ average by July 14 Baseline: Ds or less	Monitoring of attendance Set schedule of study times

> *Clinical Supervision*
>
> A clinical supervisor carefully reviews the treatment plan to be sure that it clearly validates the problem areas and impairments in a measurable and objective manner. It should match the client's presenting problem and diagnosis. Check that each objective is measurable in a manner in which the client's progress can be evaluated, and that the outcomes of therapy are apparent. Vague treatment plans lead to vague outcomes. As treatment progresses the supervisor asks for treatment plan updates and evaluates the progress of therapy. Then cases are reviewed to help determine what revisions should be made in both treatment, and in the treatment plan, to best meet the client's goals.

PROGRESS NOTES

Progress notes are the only evidence that the treatment plan is being followed. They provide a session-by-session account of the client's current conduction, ongoing stressors and impairments, progresses, treatments, referrals, and any other factors of the client's treatment. There are a number of ways to write progress notes (e.g., Subjective Objective Assessment Plan [SOAP], Data Assessment Plan [DAP]). The format of the progress notes is not as important as the content. Overall, progress notes should reflect current and ongoing progresses, setbacks, effects of specific treatments, client quotes, test results, level of cooperation, affective observations, nonverbal observations, and any other factors affecting treatment.

The following example is of a DAP progress note. The acronym DAP stands for *data assessment plan,* in which the DAP is the outline for each progress note. Progress notes will cover some of the information listed, but not every item every time.

Document every instance of client or collateral contact or missed appointments in a progress note. For example, every time a client phones you, for whatever reason, make a notation of the contact in the progress notes, whether or not it is a billable service.

Data

1. What content or topics were discussed in the session?
2. How did the session address treatment plan objectives?
3. What therapeutic interventions and techniques were employed, and how effective were they?
4. What clinical observations (behavioral, affective, etc.) were made?
5. What progress or setbacks occurred?
6. What signs and symptoms of the diagnosis are present, increasing, decreasing, or no longer present?
7. How are the treatment plan goals and objectives being met at this time?
8. What is the current medical necessity for services?
9. What is being done outside the session?
10. What are the client's current limitations and strengths?

Assessment

1. Effects or results of the current session.
2. Therapeutic progression.
3. Client's level of cooperation/insight/motivation.
4. Client progress and setbacks.
5. Areas requiring more clinical work.
6. Effectiveness of treatment strategies.
7. Completion of treatment plan objectives.
8. Changes needed to keep therapy on target.
9. Need for diagnostic revisions.

Plan

1. Homework assignments.
2. Upcoming interventions.
3. Content of future sessions.
4. Treatment plan revisions.
5. Referrals.

Example of DAP Progress Note

Name Drew Lindstrom   Chart # 0705055   Date 5-5-07

DATA: Drew arrived at the session 15 minutes late. The initial plan for the session was to role-play various situations in which she wants to be more assertive. However, when she entered the session she stated, "This is the worst week of my life. . . . I missed another three days of work and lost my job." She states that she is severely depressed and stressed about now being unemployed and having several bills to pay. She further notes that she feels very hopeless about her future. She vented several emotions, describing much frustration, anger, and feelings of rejection. We discussed her negative thought patterns, how they bring her down, and how they prevent her from believing that she can do anything about her situation. She cried several times during the session. We worked on a list of options she can consider, and emphasized positive versus negative consequences for each potential action. She stated that she will try to consider many options during the week, when she feels hopeless. Role-played asking her employer for her job back. Client was assured that she may phone the clinic or after-hours number when she feels hopeless or suicidal.

ASSESSMENT: She is very despondent and depressed about current stressors. Her level of depression has increased significantly since last session due to losing her job. Concerns are noted regarding her level of hopelessness and self-defeating thoughts.

PLAN: Reinstate sessions on biweekly basis. Continue focusing on means of analyzing negative thought patterns and feelings of hopelessness. She will contact her ex-employer within 2 days. Plus, she will apply for at least two jobs.

	Starting	Ending	
Next Appt: 5-8-07 at 2:00 P.M.	time: 2:15 P.M.	time: 3:00 P.M.	Type: 90846
Signature Helen Lockery, MA, LICSW			Date: 5-5-07

PRIMER FOR DOCUMENTING SUICIDAL/HOMICIDAL BEHAVIOR

Clinical supervisors and therapists must be well trained in both handling and documenting suicidal and homicidal behavior. Besides the obvious potential tragedy of a suicide or homicide, there can be legal ramifications for the therapist and the clinic if a client's suicidal behavior is not handled with extreme care.

Crisis management and handling suicidal behavior are a must in the training and employment orientation for clinical staff. Never assume that a therapist is trained to deal with a crisis or suicide. The clinic should have clear policies, procedures, and training to coordinate efforts.

Whenever the client suggests any issues with suicidal or homicidal behavior it is necessary to document exactly what was said, and determine the level of risk. A common taxonomy of degrees of suicide is as follows:

1. *Suicidal/homicidal ideations:* Thoughts about death or suicide or homicide. Risk can range from mild to severe.

Suicide: *"What would it be like if I wasn't around?"*

Homicide: *"I often think about getting him out of my life for good."*

2. *Suicidal threats:* Verbalizing suicidal or homicidal intent. Risk can range from mild, such as attention-seeking behavior, to severe, in cases of a serious warning given. All threats must be taken seriously.

Suicide: *"If she doesn't survive, I'm going to kill myself."*

Homicide: *"If he doesn't leave us alone, I'll put him out of his misery."*

3. *Suicidal gestures:* Suicidal or homicidal-like behaviors. Risk can range from moderate, such as a slight cut on the wrist, to severe, such as walking out into traffic.

Suicide: *"If I take any more pills that will be it."*

Homicide: *"The next time I hurt him, he'll never get up."*

4. *Suicidal plan:* An intended course of action to commit suicide. Risk is serious.

Suicide: *"When I leave here, I am going to drive to the George Washington Bridge and jump off. No one can stop me."*

Homicide: *"I'm going to kill him when he gets home. And I mean it."*

5. *Suicide attempt:* An action in which death is the goal. Risk is extreme.

Both: Drug overdose, shotgun wound.

Therapists should receive staff training that includes clear examples of each level of suicide threat. No matter what level, or nonexistence, of suicidal behavior, always document that the question about suicidality has been presented to the client. It is my opinion that not asking every client about suicidality borders on malpractice. During clinical training provide ample room for discussion on how to determine that a client is at risk for suicide.

Typically when there is a plan for suicide or homicide, and sometimes lesser levels of suicidal behavior, it is mandatory to report the potential threat. Different municipalities and organizations have different reporting rules, but a safe procedure is as follows:

1. Even when a client does not appear suicidal or homicidal, or endorses related symptoms, document that you presented questions to rule out suicidal behavior. Clearly document specific statements of denial.

2. If the client endorses any level of suicidal or homicidal behavior, specifically inquire and document the statements made. The greater the level on the taxonomy (1–5) listed previously, the greater level of documentation and client care required.

3. If the client endorses concerns such as ideations, threats, or gestures, be sure to specifically ask and document the response to questions such as, "Do you have a plan for suicide/homicide?" If there is a plan, you are mandated to report it.

4. If there is not a stated plan, clearly document the client's statements, but explain how to obtain help if problems escalate. Provide and document the resources you made available to the client.

Suicide

5. If the client has a plan for suicide, make all efforts to keep the client in your office while family and authorities are notified. I contact (1) their stated emergency contact, (2) local social service, (3) local police, and (4) the emergency room of the local hospital. To some this is excessive—however, not everyone notified will respond in a timely manner. Document each phone call or attempted phone call.

6. Make all efforts to arrange for the client to go to the emergency room at a hospital that handles psychiatric emergencies. Possible transportation could be an ambulance, the police, or a relative. However, sometimes relatives or friends do not take the client to the hospital. Validate what times each action was taken, in such a manner that it is apparent you took all precautions to protect the client's safety.

Homicide

7. If the client has a plan for homicide, immediately contact the police and the intended victim. The police should come and escort the client. Document all procedures, phone calls, and actions. If you are not able to contact the intended victim, clearly document all actions taken in the attempt (including providing the information to the police).

SURVIVING AN AUDIT

Clearly the best way to survive any type of audit is to have your patients' records in order at all times. This task is especially difficult in a mental health clinic with several therapists. Each therapist has a different level of knowledge and experience in documentation. Newer therapists may have been used to a different system, or no system, of documentation. Thus, the adage "An ounce of prevention is worth a pound of cure" unmistakably applies to an audit.

The best preparation for an audit is to always be prepared, with or without notice. In a well-managed clinic, charts are up to date as a matter of standard procedure. Audits do not have to be a time when everyone is rushing to make their charts in compliance.

This involves strict, informative management; regular staff training, and ongoing reviews of charts. When therapists are hired, be very clear that they are required to keep their paperwork up to date, and that it must be written in a standardized format that others in the clinic use. Provide them with examples of well-documented charts, and be available to them to help when they have questions.

When you interview new therapists be very clear as to the documentation guidelines and clinical standards of the clinic. Some therapists will not come to work at your clinic with these restrictions, but these are likely the same people whose documentation would lead to problems in an audit.

Charts must have an outside criterion, by which the therapist knows what is expected. Concepts such as "medical necessity" must be considered for every chart. For example, in a case review meeting, do not simply ask the supervisee if services are medically necessary, but rather, ask the supervisee to show you where in the chart medical necessity is documented. Then, go to the chart and play the devil's advocate, stating that services are not medically necessary. Require that the supervisee can demonstrate the need for services through what is already written down. An auditor will not allow you to verbally defend a case. *If it is not written down, it does not exist.*

This same method may also be used when planning treatment and writing progress notes. Ask the supervisee questions by referencing specific progress notes, and ask where the progress note indicates concepts such as current level of functioning, stressors, validation of the current diagnosis, evaluation of progress on treatment plan objectives, effects of specific treatment strategies, and the plan for the next session.

> *Example of Not Being Ready for an Audit*
> *Leading to Fraudulent Documentation*
>
> I once worked at a clinic where it was announced that there would be an audit in 2 weeks. Some of the therapists who were behind in their paperwork rushed to make their charts complete. One therapist quickly wrote a number of generic progress notes to catch up with charts that were weeks behind. Some of the same notes were placed in different clients' files, and only the names and dates were changed. The auditor quickly noticed that many of the progress notes in the therapist's charts were identical, with only the names and dates changed! It was not surprising the rest of this therapist's charts were audited, resulting in a large payback of funds to the insurance company, and the dismissal of the employee.

Before the Auditor Comes

Typically an audit is announced at least a week or more in advance. Do your best to make that date available on the calendar so that you or a specified contact person are available at all times to the auditor.

Be sure to have the charts in order prior to the audit, but do not modify information in the charts. For example, if some are missing information such as discharge summaries, catch up on that type of information. But, if information such as treatment plans and progress notes is missing or incomplete, it could be fraudulent to fill in such information, because it would likely be contrived for the sake of the audit. It is considered fraudulent to add information to existing progress notes.

When the Auditor Comes

Always be courteous to a records auditor. This person is likely a mental health professional simply doing his or her job. Let the auditor know who the contact person in the clinic will be, and keep it to that person. Do your best to make the auditor comfortable in a separate, private room, with all amenities for comfort. Unless there are ethical concerns regarding privacy issues, provide the auditor

Example of What an Auditor Checks When Reviewing a File

Clinic/Practice _____   Therapist _____

Chart Number _____

0—Not in compliance/Not in existence
1—Fair or infrequent compliance
2—Satisfactory compliance

Date of Review _____

3—Superior compliance

Reviewer _____

	0	1	2	3
1. Entries are legible	0	1	2	3
2. Records are uniformly organized	0	1	2	3
3. Testing data present	0	1	2	3
4. Testing results communicated to patient	0	1	2	3
5. Signed HIPAA compliance present	0	1	2	3
6. Rationale documented for ongoing services	0	1	2	3
7. Intake present	0	1	2	3
8. Presenting problem	0	1	2	3
9. Initial diagnosis present	0	1	2	3
10. Rationale/evidence for diagnosis	0	1	2	3
11. Treatment plan present	0	1	2	3
12. Description of impairments	0	1	2	3
13. Support for medical necessity	0	1	2	3
14. Treatment recommendations/rationale	0	1	2	3
15. Treatment addresses impairments	0	1	2	3
16. Treatment goals are attainable/realistic	0	1	2	3
17. Treatment objectives are observable/measurable	0	1	2	3
18. Client collaboration in treatment plan	0	1	2	3
19. Rationale for number of visits	0	1	2	3
20. Treatment plan follows intake material	0	1	2	3
21. Discharge criteria indicate reduction in impairments	0	1	2	3
22. Medication changes noted	0	1	2	3
23. Progress notes present	0	1	2	3
24. Progress notes dated and signed	0	1	2	3
25. Progress notes follow treatment plan objectives	0	1	2	3
26. Progress notes follow treatment plan interventions	0	1	2	3
27. Reason for termination indicated	0	1	2	3
28. Treatment outcomes described	0	1	2	3
29. Documentation of follow-up	0	1	2	3
30. Multidisciplinary review of case	0	1	2	3

0–25   Not in compliance   Subtotals ___ ___ ___ ___

26–45   Infrequent compliance

46–70   Satisfactory compliance   Total (add subtotals) ____/90

71–90   Good/Superior compliance

Comments _____

_____

with any information that is asked. Typically, you will be asked for specific files. Some files may be random, while others may have been flagged due to excessive sessions or other reasons.

When the Audit Is Over

Typically, results of an audit are not relayed to a clinic for up to several weeks. The auditor sends a packet with an explanation of results. If the purpose of the audit was educational (hopefully for the

---

The Responsibility of the Clinic Director or Supervisor

It is the clinical supervisor's responsibility to train therapists and monitor their files to protect from clinical deficiencies areas such as billing errors, inappropriate treatment, unnecessary services, and excessive services. Auditors check for these same concerns. When a therapist is hired and follows the procedures of the clinic, you have a valuable employee. When therapists do not follow the basic rules of accountability, they are potentially placing the clients, the clinic, and themselves in jeopardy. Thus, the supervisor's job involves much more than having a high level of clinical expertise. Management skills, including the ability to train, monitor, supervise, promote, and fire employees are necessary to stabilize all involved.

It is suggested that if therapists at your clinic are paid on a commission, that their contract contain a clause concerning payback of funds stemming from an audit. Make provisions in the contract that even if the files have been signed off by a clinical supervisor, but do not pass an outside audit, the therapist is ultimately responsible for the content of the files. Typically, when a payback is requested, the therapists are required to pay back the amount they received in commission. That is, if there is a $100 payback, and the therapist is paid a 55 percent commission, the therapist is liable for $55 of the payback to the insurance company.

An audit can be threatening to a clinic. However, with adequate training and supervision in documentation, you should be successful during an audit, resulting in little or no payback. If there is a payback, take it as a learning experience to aid you in the future. If the clinic cannot afford to pay the entire amount back immediately, usually payment installments can be arranged, or future payments to the clinic can be reduced until the amount is paid off.

clinic), there will be no payback of funds; it is simply a learning process. However, it is more common that an audit from an insurance company will result in a payback of funds. In such cases, an explanation of the concerns noted in each file are listed, and as are various reasons for paying back funds to the insurance company.

The clinic director generally goes over the auditor's concerns with each therapist. Then, the therapist reviews these issues and has an opportunity to appeal. If no appeals are made, the requested amount of funds must be paid back. If you decide to appeal all or some of the decisions, carefully copy each of the files, documenting the evidence that the auditor stated was not sufficient. Never add material to file after an audit. The auditor has likely copied the entire record, or at least the problem areas.

SUMMARY

Documentation skills are a necessity in this age of accountability. Simply listing symptoms is not sufficient to warrant a diagnosis, or the medical necessity for receiving mental health services. Services are considered medically necessary if documentation provides evidence that the client's mental health condition will decline, or not return to an adequate level of mental health functioning, without medical services.

The OFAID procedure is an acronym for Onset, Frequency, Antecedents, Intensity, and Duration. It is used when validating or providing measurable symptoms and impairments of clients' problem areas. The data is used in monitoring clients' progress and setbacks during treatment, and ultimately as outcome measures at termination.

Treatment plans are likened to a contract or blueprint, as when a builder builds a house. It breaks down concerns into specific problem areas to be treated. Overall goals and specific measurable and attainable objectives are set. Then the strategies that will be used in treatment are noted. Periodic progress can be evaluated by monitoring the client's progress toward each objective. Thus, periodic changes in treatment are based on this information.

Progress notes provide evidence of the effectiveness of treatment. Data is collected by observations, client statements, and other information collected. The data is assessed, then a plan is made for future sessions, based on the data and assessment. Progress notes should correspond with the treatment plan. If not, the treatment plan should be revised to reflect the current treatment.

Clinic managers and supervisors must have expertise and be able to supervise and teach therapists to provide helpful documentation, enabling the clinic to maintain standardized procedures.

Do not wait to prepare for an audit until you know it is coming. Always have all files in order and up to date, even if you are never audited. An efficient clinic director or manager is an ongoing auditor; not for the sake of finding errors, but to increase the quality of the clinic. You would be upset if your physician did not keep records of a visit you made a few weeks ago. We must hold ourselves to the same standard.

TEST YOUR KNOWLEDGE

1. The acronym OFAID is used to

   (a) define treatment strategies in a treatment plan.

   (b) provide aid to clients.

   (c) describe various aspects of impairment.

   (d) none of these.

2. Which of the following best represents a treatment plan goal?

   (a) Alleviate depressive symptoms.

   (b) Increase social activities to three times per week.

   (c) Provide dialectical behavioral therapy (DBT).

   (d) Make a psychiatric appointment.

3. Which of the following best represents a treatment plan objective?

   (a) Alleviate depressive symptoms.

   (b) Increase social activities to three times per week.

(c) Provide DBT.

(d) Make a psychiatric appointment.

4. Which of the following best represents assessment in a DAP progress note?

(a) Client states that she phoned her mother this week.

(b) Client described much happiness about phoning her mother this week.

(c) The act of phoning her mother appears to be therapeutically helpful.

(d) Client will phone her mother this week.

5. Scrambling to get ready for an audit, such as catching up on old progress notes, according to this book, is considered

(a) unethical.

(b) a standard acceptable practice.

(c) a necessary means to avoid a high payback.

(d) none of these.

Answers: 1. c; 2. a; 3. b; 4. c; 5. a

End-of-Book Humor

Over the years I've jotted down some statements that have been made by well-meaning clients.

"I get pancake attacks."

"I have anxiety trips."

"I have backflashes."

"I have schizo-defective disorder."

"I have psycho-effective disorder."

"I have diarrhea of unknown origin."

"I have impulsivity explosive disorder."

"My long-term memory is better than my future memory."

"My extension span is poor."

"My problem is that I am mentally efficient."

"I was told to get a psychic evaluation from you."

"I was diagnosed with maniac depression."

"I have a learning disorderly."

"I have demotional problems."

"I have sleepy apnea."

"My child has opposite defisition disorder."

"My son has emotional attachment disorder."

"My son has operational defiant disorder."

"My child has a disbehavior disorder."

"I switch from hypergetic to quiet."

"I have issues to be dissolved."

"My family is splattered across the country."

"Everyday it takes me 3 days to get things done."

"Her right knee was very swallowed."

"I get disoriental."

"I had an autopsy pregnancy."

"My daughter is pregnant and she is having a baby."

"I have been in in-house and outhouse therapy."

"It's hard for me to detain information."

"He's really frittery."

"During the holidays I was a bell ringer for the savage army."

Client: "I have a long-standing problem."

Therapist: "What do you mean?"

Client: "I can't stand very long."

Client: "I was diagnosed with bipolar."

Therapist: "By whom?"

Client: "By Polar."

Previous treatment plan in client's record: "Maintain current level of symptoms of depression and anxiety."

Index

CPSIA information can be obtained at www.ICGtesting.com
Printed in the USA
LVOW03s2013300315

432627LV00009B/80/P